A Cure for the World

Your End to Pain, Forever

By

Roy Knight Jr

Damaged and Concerned Consumer

ISBN-13: 978-1544267289

ISBN-10: 1544267282

Copyright © 2017 Roy Knight Jr

All rights reserved.

ACKNOWLEDGMENTS

This would not have been possible without the research and instruction given by Dr. David Perlmutter and Dr. William Davis and Dr. Daniel Amen, The British Medical Journal, the New England Journal of Medicine, NIH's PubMed and Wikipedia also were very important in the construction of this book an important part in the construction of this book. I tried to attribute every passage used from those sources.

Credit also goes to James, for without his comments," No one even knows or cares about this".

© Wolfberry | Dreamstime.com ©Ffatserifade|Dreamstime.com - Evolution

© Alain Lacroix | Dreamstime.com - Sugar consumption

Foreword

I followed *Time for the Ultimate Cure* with *A Cure For the World* because the second book didn't even tell the whole story. Although the first two books don't complete the story, its importance is as crucial to know. The information in my first book, *It's Time For a Cure*, details 17 disorders and diseases and how they're influenced by glycation which is influenced by glucose consumption. Honestly, that was all I thought this was responsible for. Then, I looked into it deeper, and the deeper I delved into it, the bleaker the picture got. Then all of a sudden it turned ugly, really ugly.

In the second book, I found out who is responsible for most of the damage done by glycation and how they magnified the problem with their herbicide, Roundup.

This has now become a movement. This is a movement to bring back sanity and dignity to America and the world. That sanity and dignity have been stolen from us for the last thirty years. It goes back to the time when a company started dabbling in genetically modified seeds and soon earned a patent for a creation of nature, a seed. This is a story of a for-profit chemical corporation and their political engineering of our government, to assume control over government agencies, and the desire of that corporation to completely control our food supply. With the help of some strategic placements in the Supreme Court and certain gov't agencies, this corporation has succeeded in acquiring unprecedented control over the food we eat and what that creates. What it creates in itself, is devastating.

The only way to stop the destruction that this industry is responsible for is to stop buying their products until they decide to change them and give us something healthier to eat. *It's Time For A Cure!* The world must know what is being done to them without their consent or knowledge.

To make this volume easier to read, I suggest that you scan through the PubMed reports unless one applies to your situation. If that's the case, hopefully, it will help you to clarify your condition and to heal you. Because healing is what it's all about, not continuing treatment, but healing.

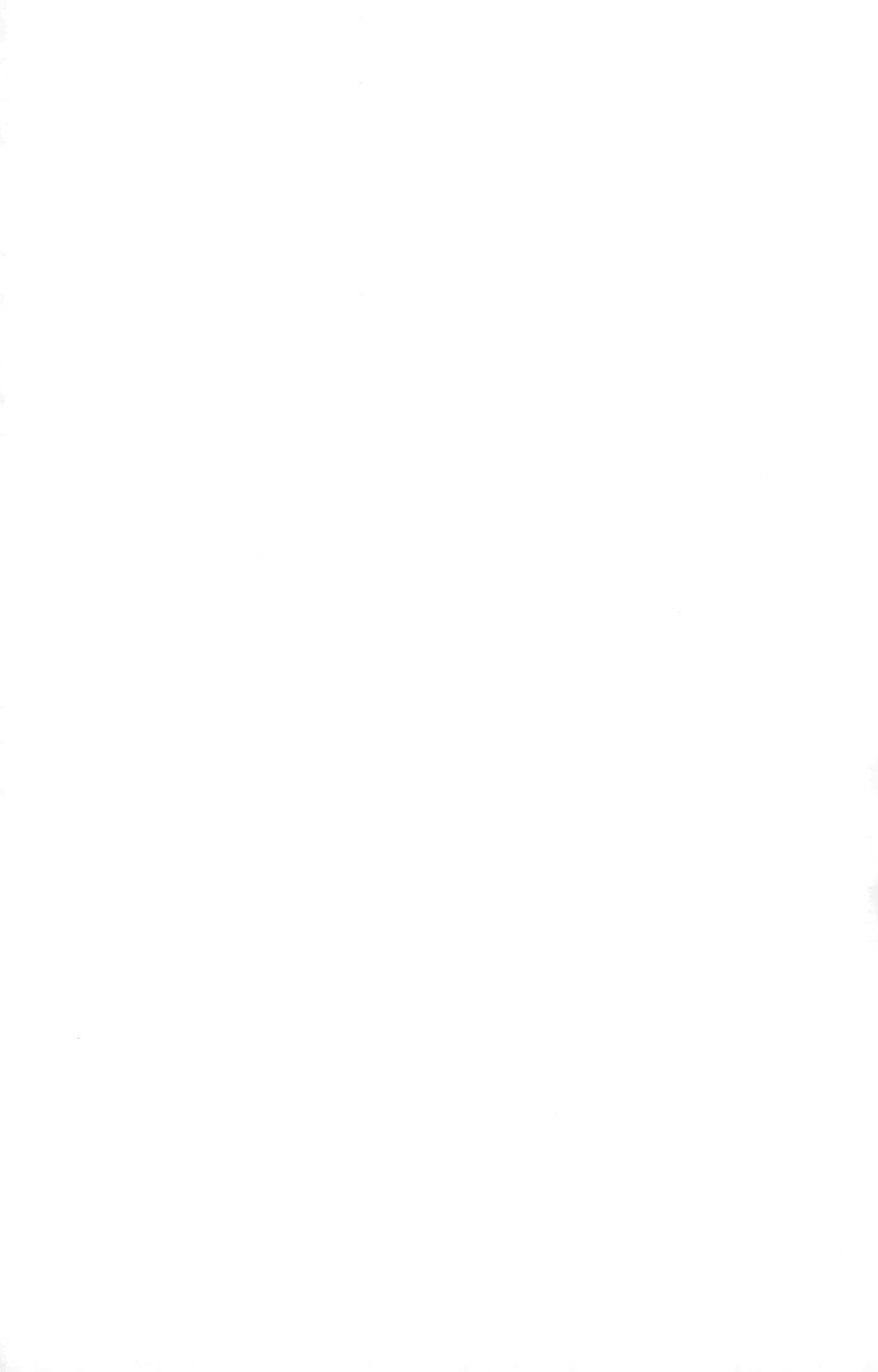

Part I Danger Lurks in your Food

1	My Whole Wheat Story	Pg10
2	New Dangers Of Grain Consumption Due To Continued Contamination By Glyphosate Herbicides	Pg21
3	The Glyphosate Poisoning of America and the World	Pg28

Part II Enzymatic Damage

4 Calories, Do Your Worry About Them? — Pg41

5 Can Your Type of Cancer be Cured or Just Treated? — Pg50

6 Can You Type of Heart Disease Be Cured or Just Treated — Pg66

7 Can Your Dementia, Osteoporosis, IBS, IBD, Or Other Disease Of Inflammation Be Cured Or Just Treated? — Pg73

8 Understanding Why We Fight/The Best Way to Fight Hunger Fights Terrorism — Pg90

Part III The Way Forward

9 The Way Forward – Fasting And The Ketogenic Diet — Pg109

10 God's Answer — Pg122

About the Author — Pg131

PMC Report Credits — Pg132

<u>WARNING!</u>

This book provides the warnings that the FDA and the USDA won't, because of their own addiction to this food, and their association with the food industry.

Part 1

Physical Consequences of a Carbohydrate Diet

Dependence
(The Addiction)

Hunger Cycle
(Manifestation of Dependence)

Inflammation
(Manifestation of AGEs and Foundation of Pain)

Chapter 1
My Whole Wheat Story

To easier understand my thought as you read through this dialogue, I thought you should have a little more background on the author, so I included this addendum to my story.

The first thing I remember is being given a bath in the kitchen sink. I remember a yellow dinette set in our kitchenette upstairs at my foster grandparent's house in Wayne Ohio. It was my father's foster parent's house in Wayne, one of two that they had along with a furniture store across the street. The house was basically on the opposite corner of the intersection where we ended up living in Wayne. I can remember sitting down on the top stair so I could scooch down the stairs to reach the bottom because I couldn't step down each step. My legs just weren't long enough. (Scooching is sliding your butt forward on each step to fall to the next step on your butt.) This is the only way a toddler can navigate a stairway until their legs are long enough to clear each step. I can vaguely remember the day I was able to walk down the stairs and how big I felt. I can, though, remember my mother scolding me for not walking down the stairs when I was able to but didn't (it was too easy to scooch). I guess she was tired of the butt in my pants wearing out so quickly.

My father was quite possibly the only foster child where he went to school in Wayne. He started school in West Millgrove, Ohio in a two-room school with a half dozen other students in grades 1-8, then transferred to Wayne school which was a 1-12 school when he reached the ninth grade. It was here where he met my mother, who grew up on a farm, two miles north of town. Even though he was born just outside of Toledo in Millbury, Ohio, the child placement agency who put my father in a foster home after he was abandoned by his mother and his father couldn't take care of him, decided to send him 25 miles south to West Millgrove, on the other side of the county. His siblings, two sisters and a brother were born in a different county in Toledo (Lucas County), so they were sent to a different foster home, separating my father from the rest of his family. If this never happened, I wouldn't be here as Dad would have never met Mom. They met in school in Wayne where Mom was in the same grade as Dad and even though they graduated approximately 4-5 years before I was born, the school had been transformed into an elementary school by the time I attended 1st and 2nd grades there.

I can remember standing by my grandfather in his red plaid robe, working on a jigsaw puzzle. Even though I can't remember his wife, my foster grandmother very well, I can remember a vision of her standing in her kitchen downstairs in that house we first lived in after Dad returned from his Air Force service at FE Warren AFB in Cheyenne, WY, where I and my oldest sister were born. My life in Wayne started 8 months after I was born in April 1954. It ended in Wayne when we moved to Tucson, Arizona in the fall of 1962. I had just started 2nd grade. I remember my teacher's name as Mrs. Stahl.

I finished 2nd grade, 3rd grade, 4th grade in Tucson, Arizona where we became resident tourists. I loved Arizona so much, I had to return there as soon as I graduated junior college. Although I started 5th grade in Tucson, we soon moved to Albuquerque, NM where I finished 5th and 6th grades. By the time I started 7th grade we had moved to Omaha, NE, where I completed 7th and started 8th grade. Halfway through 8th grade, we moved to Urbandale, IA, a suburb of Des Moines where I also finished 9th grade. From there, we moved to Fort Dodge, IA, where I graduated from high school and Jr College.

As soon as I graduated, I left for Arizona as I fell in love with the state when we lived there while I was in Elementary School. I moved to Phoenix where my sister was living as she had moved back two years earlier. I had planned to attend ASU to further my education in music since I'd taken piano lessons most of my life and was an OK - good pianist. Even in Wayne where I started piano lessons before I started School, there was someone better than I who was about the same age as I. I think this was the start of my self-image as being inferior. It seems for the rest of my life, I was always 2nd or 3rd best and never the best. It seems that this helped to develop an attitude in my mind of my inferiority and that I'd been destined to be a loser all my life. From the self-denigrating humor I engaged in all my life to the negativity I lived with most of the time, and how I felt about minorities and most people that weren't like me, it wasn't surprising I had set myself up for failure. Too bad I didn't know any better at that time.

I met my first wife in Ft Dodge, IA where I graduated from high school and college. It was a junior college in the town where my girlfriend/fiancée's mother worked as a teacher. Her father was a county psychologist. Having parents with that kind of education was a bit out of my league. I owe my life to them, for without their help I would have never survived my high school and college. As smart as I was, I had multiple learning disabilities that did more to hold me back than anything else. I think looking back on it now, I see that I had just enough ADD to make it difficult to learn anything in a classroom setting. I had the same problem then, that I have now, once I learn something, my attention is too easily distracted, to learn something new, instead of mastering the one already learned. That's because it's easier. I graduated with a GDP that was low, very low. My GDP was low because of unrecognized learning disabilities. I see now, this was due to my diet high in carbs, fluctuating my glucose levels, unbeknownst to me. I can only imagine what Irene thought when her daughter, Jane and I left for Arizona on our honeymoon the day after we got married. All I can only say, I'm sorry,

Irene. I am truly grateful for everything you did for me throughout my school years in Ft Dodge and I failed to compensate you for your effort. If it's any consolation, I failed to repay my mother as well, before she passed. The biggest mistake in my life was when I let your daughter leave me. I didn't fight enough to keep her. She's still my soul mate, the love of my life. My greatest dismay is losing her.

I hear other people say "they'd never change anything they've done in their life." I can't say that. I've made far too many mistakes. If I could, I'd go back and change every one of them. But then, I would have to have had more foresight, which is something a 20-year-old has little of. Foresight can only be learned as it's the foundation of wisdom. I certainly could have used more of that, then.

When Jane and I landed in Phoenix, 3 days after our wedding in Iowa, we were excited and anxious to start work so we could establish residency to finish our schooling. I wanted to lower my tuition rates to the resident rates for ASU where I had planned to finish my degree in music since I'd been playing piano since the age of four, I thought my love of music could carry me through school. It possibly could have if I would have returned to school. But after working for a year, I failed to return to school. I lost sight of my goals. Worse yet, I didn't pay attention to my wife's goals. I'd like to blame it on not knowing her goals, but I have to take responsibility for that too, as I didn't ask her what her goals were. That was my bad. My decisions to keep working and not return to school laid out the pathway I would take from then on in my life and the life of my then-wife, Jane, and we both suffered because of it. I let us both down by not returning to school. I did more damage to Jane than I did to myself, as her odds of being successful were a lot greater than mine, simply because she was much smarter than I. Even though I knew it then, I was too proud to realize it consciously. That was probably why I didn't know what she wanted out of life, or what her goals were. A little foresight clearly would have prevented that regret.

Our decision to quit school came at the opportunity of low-cost housing, as we found a house for rent in north Phoenix for about the same price we were paying for our apartment in Tempe. Just 2 miles away from ASU where I wanted to continue my schooling. The house we moved to was 18-20 miles away, depending on the route we took to get back to Tempe. This move took us away from the school where we needed to be close to, to finish our education. This move virtually ended our prospects for further education. For all intents and purposes, we were dead in the water. This is where we started treading water and not getting ahead. This was also the start of the end of our relationship. From this point on, I became a loser.

I worked several jobs starting the best place I could, for an uneducated man, retail. Retail offered me an opportunity to learn how to get along with people, as retail sales is a people person's job. One thing my life had taught me was how to make friends. A life of moving from state to state transferring to different schools had taught me how to make friends and I made friends, well, very well. That would prove to be advantageous later on in my life after I lost everything as a result of injuries received in a car accident.

Making friends seemed always easy to me and that allowed me to dabble in several different areas of retail and sales, eventually leading me to a career as a life insurance agent. But since this was a career that came after the accident that's defined my life, it was more difficult to achieve. My life then has been a tale of two lives, pre-accident and post-accident.

BAD DREAM REALIZED

The last thing I remember before the accident was headlights coming at me fast enough to total the car I was riding in. The next thing I remember was that I had to get out of where I was. I was in the hospital and I didn't know why I was there. All I knew was that I didn't like hospitals or anything about them. I hated the way they smelled and the fact that's there's nothing to do in a hospital, especially if you're a patient. I didn't realize that I was a patient in the ICU. I'd learned later that they air evacuated me to St Joseph's in Phoenix, even though my fiancé had instructed the paramedics to send me to a closer hospital in Scottsdale.

They recognized that I had a head injury and sent me to St Joseph's hospital because of Barrows neurological clinic. My mother always said it was that clinic that saved my life. I don't know, I was in a coma. I have a faint memory of a formula that they fed me through my nose when I couldn't eat anything solid. I can also remember the tubes in my nose and when they pulled them out.

When I came out of the coma, I was paralyzed and didn't even know it. All I knew was that I had to get out of there, so I removed the straps around my wrists, crawled out of bed and fell flat on my ass. No one was prepared for that. I remember that I had defecated on the floor when I fell. I can remember an aide cussing about having to clean it up, along with me. My next memory was in the shower getting cleaned off. I learned the hard way about my paralysis. I thought I could walk when I couldn't even stand. I was bedridden and didn't even know it or why.

My first trip to therapy was on a gurney because I couldn't sit up in a wheelchair. I don't remember exactly when I graduated to the wheelchair, I just remember my first or second ride in it was with a tray on the arms of the chair, to support my upper body. I still couldn't sit up and needed to use the tray to lay my head on. I can remember going across a walkway from the hospital over to the rehab center every time we had to go to therapy. I can also remember yelling and swearing a lot at the therapists. Even though my mother was there all the time, she said little to nothing. All she could do was to tolerate my outbursts and scold me when it got too abusive.

This was the start of my new life. I was used to something completely different. I was used to a very active life. My biggest gripe was that I had to drive my truck to go bowling 3 times a week because I couldn't carry two or three bowling balls on either of my bikes. I rode my motorcycles a lot. Everyone thought the accident I was in, happened while I was on my bike, because of my head injury. (That's what I get for riding without a helmet all of the time.)

I was bowling so much because I thought I might be able to go professional. My average was 186 and bowled on two scratch teams. I needed to maintain an average of 205 to go pro and was practicing as much as I could to achieve that goal. Instead of saving my earnings, I invested them in my future, using the excuse of practicing, to do something I enjoyed immensely, like bowling.

My golf game was a different story. My best golf game was a 93 on a 7600 + yd course. I usually play the par 3's though because I always seemed to like to take the scenic route around the course, every time I golfed. If I was going to be good at golf, it would have taken way too long to be prosperous, so I stuck with the bowling.

That was until I decided to further my education by getting a degree or diploma in electronics. That was four months before the life-changing accident happened. My plans to change my life for the better had been put on hold...for how long was anyone's guess.

What I was about to find out was that the "how long" was going to be forever. My life still hasn't gotten any better. I've had to struggle more than most to achieve what I've had through life. Even though my life is yet to get better, my recovery has just started taking off, thanks to my change in diet.

Where I'm at now is a far cry from where I was when I came out of my coma. When you look at me now, you can't tell that I'm paralyzed. You can't even see it when I walk. You can only see it when I run or attempt to do anything athletic. And I used to be an athlete. I was a runner, a distance runner. I wish I knew then what I know now, how much better a diet of fat is to that of carbs. I could have saved myself a lot of grief just by following a different diet.

Now, since my disability is invisible, my biggest problem is that my disability is unrecognizable to the naked eye. I've perfected my appearance as much as I can, to make myself appear normal. The problem is, it takes a lot of effort just to maintain that illusion still, even with my improved health. But from laying around and doing little more than watch TV, this new ability I've gained to put my thought into print has given me a new life. If I could only instruct my fingers to stop fat-fingering" everything I type, my life would be able to move forward much easier. But that's part of my disability and I guess everyone with a disability has to work slower, but I don't appear like I should have to. I look completely normal and only those who know me closely know of my disabilities.

That has a tendency to create questions in people's minds about what kind of a person I really am since they see a completely normal person, but underneath has severe handicaps that keep me from functioning properly. I can only function haphazardly at best, because of the effort it takes just to appear normal. Fortunately, most people are more patient than I. But then, almost all others don't have the brain damage that I get to live with. Thus, the crux of my disability, the inability to see it, making my disability invisible if not completely invisible to the naked eye.

My days of selling life insurance came shortly after GMO seeds emerged from the laboratories at Monsanto. (Their success in patenting this new type of seed would later have deadly consequences on the public and their health and eventually take its toll on their minds.) My career selling life insurance didn't last more than 10 years because of the result of a second car accident that gave me a hernia. I was coming home from taking my wife to work across town when a car ran a red light to broadside my car while traveling somewhere around 40-45 MPH. The car was totaled and I suffered a hernia along with a knock on the noggin from the passenger side mirror after breaking through the passenger's window. I also suffered whiplash that still gives me pain today.

This was the second severe accident I've been a victim of. On December 24 at 00:00 hrs a drunk driver ran a red light and broadsided the car my fiancé was driving to put me in a come for a month, with a severe closed head injury. That head injury prompted two massive strokes which nearly took my life. Whether fortunate or unfortunate, I lived. When I came out of the coma I was completely paralyzed. I felt like a fly on flypaper except that I couldn't move at all. My first trip to therapy was on a gurney. Quite possibly my second trip was also.

When I graduated to a wheelchair, they had to put a tray on the chair to support my upper body because I didn't have the strength to hold my upper body upright. Even though it's a vague memory I can remember my head laying down on the tray while in the wheelchair. I can also remember shouting and swearing at the therapists for what they were putting me through, but if they didn't put me through all that, I wouldn't be where I am today. I was literally a basket case, at best. The doctors told my family that I might have a 50-50 chance of survival, considering the injuries I sustained.

Because I was used to working all my life, my first goal was to get back to work, so I found the only work I could do, sitting and watching, as a security guard. Well, this job also involved walking around but I had relearned to walk by then, so I could handle at least that much. I just couldn't do much of anything else. (It's a good thing I didn't have to chase anyone.) All of my other skills were thrown out the window with my brain injury and subsequent strokes. Have you ever had a massive stroke? They're life changing, to say the least. I had two of them within a 30 minute period. This is what brought me to the brink of death on 12/24/1984.

They leave you with nothing but a shell of a body to work with and the shell you're left with can't function properly either, so you're stuck, like a fly on flypaper. There's not much you can do about it except years and years of therapy. By the time that's through, your life has been changed so much that you're in a whole new world that's never going to revert to your old normal one. The one you have now is so different (due to your lack of abilities that you're used to living with), all you can do is adapt and learn how to live again. This is very time-consuming. Regardless of what you had learned or been through prior to any injuries, your total focus is to return to your prior prowess.

Although this assumes that you had any prowess in the first place, it's safe to assume that I did have some, at least. At the age of 26, I owned my own home, had a successful career which I was in the process of changing, successfully at age 30. I was starting my own construction company, which I followed up on, later in my life,

I'm still trying to figure out why I'm still alive. For the most part of the past 30 years, I've languished in pain and loss of function, to the point that I still have problems with balance, coordination, reasoning, judgment and most of all residual weakness on my right side, the side that was paralyzed from the strokes. As much as I try to rid my body of those detriments, I can't. They're stuck with me for the rest of my life and there is nothing I can do about it except to accept it. That may be the hardest thing to live with and subsequently brought me to my search to regain some of my lost abilities. I had been told that I'd never regained them as brain cells don't grow back.

At least that's what I thought until I read Dr. Perlmutter's book *Grain Brain*. His book taught me that the brain damage I suffered wasn't at all permanent. He also taught me that a lot of the damage to my brain, I was doing myself, with my diet. I had always thought that brain cells couldn't grow back once they were lost. I was wrong; they can grow back in many parts of the brain. This gave me hope that what I have lost 32 years prior, might be brought back. I might be able to regain some of the intelligence that I had lost from the accident and ensuing coma and strokes. This is when I changed my diet and started to bring those lost cells back. I did it initially by stopping my bread intake. Subsequently, I've ended all carbohydrate consumption and I have no intentions of going back. The glucose just does too much damage to the body to be worth its little bit of energy.

Pre-accident I was smart but uneducated. This was because of my learning disabilities, ADHD. When I was a kid, ADHD was considered just a "rambunctious kid", a daydreaming kid who couldn't keep his mind on what he was doing because it became too boring. Today this is defined as ADHD, so what I live with now, is ADD. Actually, I like to call it AAADD, Age Attributive Attention Disorder. Mine's been magnified by my disability, brain damage from a severe closed head injury that should have left me an invalid forever. My decline would be continuing if it weren't for Dr. Perlmutter's book *Grain Brain*. His book recommended to try his Keto diet and after going carb free two years earlier, it seemed a good idea.

The carb-free life did wonders for me but the keto diet is what's brought my mental abilities back along with some added, coordination returned to my right side, something I didn't expect. I explain how this has happened in my first book in the article on *Life without carbs*. Actually, I touch on it in several articles. It has to do with the effects that Ghrelin has on your body and the advantages of being Ghrelin resistant, instead of Leptin resistant, the condition of most carboholics. This is the sign of addiction. It was an addiction that I lived with for 59 years.

That's given me 59 years of damage that this food has done to my body. The plaque that I created in those 59 years still flows through my blood. It may until I die. That's a form of glycation that may not ever disappear. That means I made a wise decision to stop eating what was creating it. My health has only improved since I made that decision.

I mentioned earlier that I had lost everything from that car accident that put me in the coma, actually, I had thought I had lost everything, that was until I was in another accident 9 years later that left me with an inguinal hernia that has since left me with more problems since the repair surgery than prior. That's where my chronic severe pain comes from. The hernia repair left me with a damaged nerve trapped in scar tissue that's still creating pain today.

That drove me to a life on Oxycontin, Morphine, Oxycodone; the list goes for 23 different pain medications and anti-depressants which did little for me except to make me fat, lazy and stupid. Stupid I was for continuing that lifestyle. I didn't know what drove that lifestyle until I gave up bread. Breaking that addiction was the start of a whole new life for me. I was truly born again. No carboholic can ever know this. You have to give up the addiction to know it. But once you know it, you'll never go back to your old life of a glucose diet. (I've since learned that this is the best way to control that pain.)

That was post second accident. That's the one that has disabled me completely for 20+ years, mostly because of the drugs I was taking to manage the pain. These drugs did more to worsen my health, than my previous life of 40 years of carb ingestion had done to it. I can see now, the dependence I had in my addiction to glucose at that time. More than that, I can feel the effects of that dependence that I had on sugar (including bread). The effects of that dependence (addiction) are being felt now every time I get out of bed in the morning or whenever I nap. My back doesn't want me to move. It would rather that I stay in bed and not put any weight on it,

That's due to the degenerative disk disease I live with, in my lower back.

That is directly due to the diet of bread that my mother raised me in my whole life. That was because that's what she was raised on. That's what my family, going back as far as I can track, was raised on. This addiction goes back to the dawn of history when man first started farming this grain, Because of that this addiction has been with us forever and that's why it's so impossible to see when you're in it. But then nobody sees addictions they have, especially if that addiction was imposed upon them without their knowledge, which is exactly the problem of today's addiction. (Because they add sugar to baby food, anyone who's been fed baby food has been fed sugar. And if you've been fed sugar as a baby, you've had enough to be addicted. Try to remember the last day you didn't need to eat. That is a cycle you are addicted to. It's a dependence on a diet. What my new diet has taught me is a diet of sugar and carbs is a diet that needs to be re-fed every 2 or 3 hours. This is the nature of a carb diet, where the keto diet doesn't have any cycles. You're free from the glucose cycle of hunger and satiety. The problem is that I didn't learn this until three years ago.

So all this time, I was sabotaging my own life with my cycles of destruction, while I was on a carb diet. I never realized that until I changed my diet to a keto diet. Because of my emotional cycles, I went through several jobs. That gave me the varied experiences I needed, to see the picture that I'm putting together in this *It's Time for a Cure* series.

This carb diet that I led my life with, not only damaged my professional life, it damaged beyond repair, my body. It damaged my professional career by making me live my life within the cycle of hunger. You know what that cycle leads to. That's a cycle that leads to most other destructive cycles, as explained in Fighting Hunger Fights Terrorism Also, it's because it's caused by the hormonal action tied to your hunger cycle and it has a tendency to be destructive because it drives greed.

I can say this because I was in that world when I was on my carbohydrate diet when I was addicted to glucose. It's something you never see until you break the addiction and that why I didn't realize it for 60 years. Being raised on bread and pasta and cereal, I lived on bread and pasta and cereal all my life, up until 3 years ago. That was when the change started. It's continuing with these books. It will continue with my foundation, Save Your Dignity.

That is a far cry from where I was 32 years ago, laying in a coma with a 50/50 chance of survival. What's remarkable is my recovery cycle. It was completely stagnant on a carb diet. It wasn't until I went low-carb diet and quit eating bread and pasta and cereal and everything that was breaded, that my health started to improve. The best part is it improved without medication and it automatically came with weight loss. I had quit all of the meds 9 years earlier when I started exercising.

I've always exercised, all my life, on and off. Ever since I could walk, I've loved to run. So when I landed at St Jo's hospital by helicopter and they examined me for my injuries, 32 years ago, they saw by my brain scans that there were bruises on my brain that were creating swelling within my cranium. They had to put shunts in my skull to release the pressure. They told my parents that I would probably be a vegetable for the rest of my life and that they'd probably have to take care of me.

Fortunately for me, they encouraged me to stay in my home with my fiancée, we had just gotten engaged the night of the accident. We got married shortly after I was released from the hospital. The marriage lasted approximately 5 years. It was a marriage of love and hate, arguments, and lovemaking. It was a marriage of cycles tied to our glucose addictions. And we were addicted big time. That's why we argued as much as we did, and we love to argue. That's because we loved our carbs, in spades. We were both skinny as bean poles, so we could eat this food without consequence, at least to our waistlines, while in our 20's. The weight comes usually in the 30's, but it's been coming earlier lately. That's due to the GMO.

3 years ago, I decided to stop eating bread and everything else that the grain wheat was in. I didn't realize at that time, how this was going to manifest, but it turned out to be the best decision I have ever made. I have never been happier about making that decision. My health has improved steadily ever since I made that decision. What's most important, it continues to improve on a daily basis, and the best part is it's improving my brain's power. That's exactly the answer I've been searching for, for 30 years.

Thank you, Dr. Perlmutter!

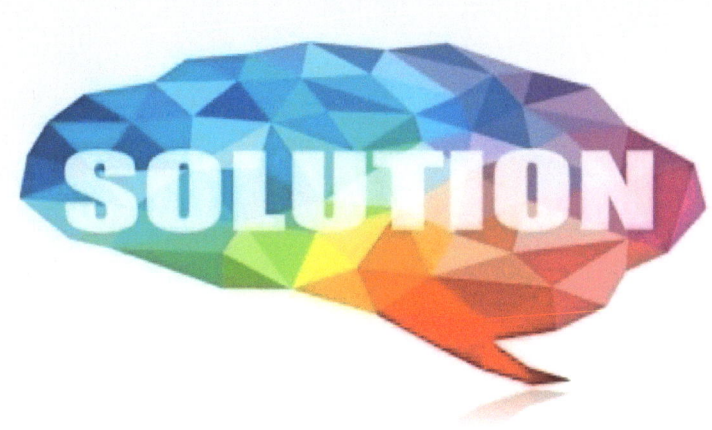

Part I

THE DANGER LURKING IN YOUR FOOD

CHAPTER 2
NEW DANGERS OF GRAIN CONSUMPTION DUE TO CONTINUED CONTAMINATION BY GLYPHOSATE HERBICIDES

You know what Roundup is don't you? Would you drink it if you could? Probably not, I least, I wouldn't. Would you eat something that it's been drowned in it? If you knew what it was, you probably wouldn't touch that either.

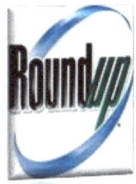

Do you realize that every bite of bread you take, you're eating Roundup, a glyphosate, enzyme inhibiting herbicide? Every corn chip you eat, you're eating glyphosate with it, also. It's in the nature of how this herbicide is used on all the grains it's sprayed on, and how it affects your body when you eat those grains. And you eat those grains every day in massive amounts. That should concern you more than anything else. Everything hinges on your health, if it's not the best, you're not your best.

This is something the food industry doesn't want you to know because it's the warning about genetically modified crop seed that's ready to accept the Roundup herbicide that kills all the weeds that rob the crops of their room to grow. This Roundup is a glyphosate herbicide responsible for inhibiting how enzymes work. That's how it kills weeds. That's also how it makes you sick. That means that the pharmaceutical industry doesn't want you to know either. Their survival depends on your pain, which is dependent on your consumption of these grains. (Monsanto found a way to ramp up that need 30 years ago when they formulated Roundup.) They inhibit enzymes that create senescence in plants. This also creates senescence in your body by inhibiting the same enzymes in your bodies. This has created a far greater need in pharmaceuticals leading to their record profits.

How sick it makes you, depends on how much of it you eat and how fast you eat it. If you eat any of the grains that this herbicide is sprayed on, you will experience future illness. The enzyme inhibiting glyphosate will see to that. The amount you ingest with each bite is so minute that you'll never notice the damage until it's too late. By that time, you'll be a slave to the pharmaceutical industry. Good luck then. Their only goal is to treat you, not cure you. Cures don't guarantee return customers, only treatment can do that.

Glucose, which used to be called glycose, is the sugar form of glycerin or glycerol. (Glycerol is a sweet lipid used for sweetening.) It's healthier than the sugar, because it's slower in satiating, and not as sweet as glucose or fructose, but that's beside the point. The point here is that fat (lipids) is healthier than carbs to eat. This points to why it's better for your body to make its own glucose instead of cholesterol, which is what it does when you feed it carbs and sugar. That's why eating only protein and fat is healthier for the body, as it allows the body to create its own glucose instead of feeding it that dirty glucose you get from carbs. Every time you eat carbs, you're getting dirty glucose at best. It's not only dirty, it's polluted with a carcinogenic glyphosate herbicide, called Roundup.

Farmers spray the Roundup on their crops to kill them, about two weeks before harvest, so they'll dry out quicker. This practice is called desiccating and it's a common practice in northern climates where the environment is a little damper like it is in North Dakota, the nation's largest wheat producer, where this is practiced on a regular basis. This is news that is not good. This news means that a good majority of bread and pasta that you eat has had Roundup sprayed on it within two weeks of harvesting, simply so the harvesting will go quicker. This puts more money in the pockets of farmers due to quicker turnover, but it puts most of the extra cash in Monsanto's pockets by selling more Roundup. It's easy to see now, how 2.6 billion pounds of it were sprayed in the US alone, in the last 20 years. What you need to do is consider how this may affect your health and if there is anything you can do about it.

According to **Natural Society's** website; Most heavily Glyphosate sprayed grains;

Roundup, the very same Monsanto-made product which contains the recently-declared carcinogenic chemical glyphosate (along with inert ingredients that are also extremely dangerous), is sprayed on your food just weeks to months before you eat it.

Which Crops Exactly? Monsanto **recommends spraying for**:

Wheat, Oats, Non-GMO Canola, Flax, Peas, Lentils, Non-GMO Soybeans, Dry Beans, Sugar Cane.

That amounts to just about every grocery store food you can think of – after all, what **DOESN'T** contain wheat, oats, soy, or sugar cane just for starters?

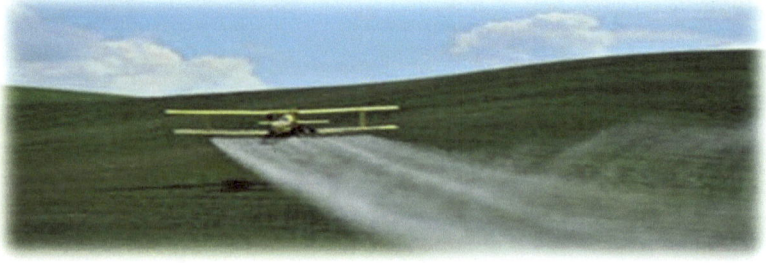

What grains do you eat, cereal grains or legume grains? (Do you like beans like I did. I was raised on them.) It really doesn't matter. They're all been doused over and over again with the glyphosate herbicide, Roundup. Do you eat sugar? You should already know how bad sugar is for you. I guess Monsanto didn't think it was bad enough. They want to make it more dangerous. Even cane sugar gets desiccated before harvest. Why?

They claim it's to help farmers. It's really to sell more Roundup. My guess is it has something to do with their involvement in the pharmaceutical industry. Having owned Searle pharmaceuticals and being merged with Pharmacia less than twenty years ago, it leaves little doubt in my mind why they're motivated to continue this deadly ruse. I know where their investments were, so I have a good idea of where they are.

The only unfortunate thing about this ruse is, you're the victim of it by buying into it. That means every time you buy your corn chips, you're buying into this ruse. It's a ruse to control your appetite by controlling your hunger. It's basically pretty simple. Whenever you eat any kind of grain it breaks down to its simplest form in your body, and that's glucose. Glucose regulates your hunger. Glucose does this by controlling your hormones, which in turn, control your emotions, with hunger just being one of them.

What most people don't realize is that hunger is just as much an emotion as fear or anger. Incidentally, fear and anger are both controlled by hunger. So are composure and sobriety. Those emotions are much higher on the tone scale than fear and anger, though. This only shows the danger of the hunger cycle and the emotions it controls.

That all points to the fact that if you can control hunger you can control everything it controls. So how do you control hunger? To control hunger you must control that which creates hunger. There's one thing in your diet that influences hunger more than anything else. That one thing is sugar.

Sugar influences your hunger by playing with your hormones, Leptin and Ghrelin first and foremost. Leptin is your satiety hormone. It tells you when you're full and to stop eating. Ghrelin, on the other hand, is your hunger hormone. It makes your stomach growl when your sugar levels get low. This is the secret to controlling hunger. Control your sugar levels and you can control your hunger. Sounds simple, doesn't it?

It is simple. It's just not that easy. But it's vital to accomplishing this step if you want to control your hunger. That means that you should eliminate as many grain foods as possible for this task to be accomplished. This will have multiple benefits for your health.

1. It will cut down on most all glycation that takes place in your body.
2. It will reduce the number of glyphosate herbicides that you ingest with every bite you take of your bagel, croissant or sandwich. (all sandwiches are contaminated)
3. It will reduce the extra glycation that the glyphosate creates
4. It will keep you off of future drug needs

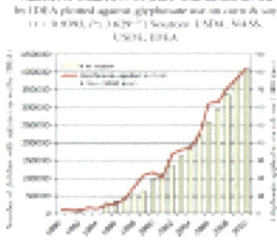

5. That will save you tons of dollars in medical costs meaning no more;
6. Treatments
7. Therapy
8. Surgery
9. Time wasted in doctors' offices reading magazines that you'd never read in the first place

Don't you have enough things to do? Can you really afford to spend that much time in a doctor's office waiting for treatment or a prescription for your pain? I used to spend half of my day dealing with doctors. Going to the appointment, waiting to see the doctor or therapist at the appointment, then waiting for more at the pharmacy for the prescription I was given to treat my pain. Notice that I mentioned, treat. That's all doctors do anymore. They're there to treat your pain not cure it. Curing it would mean that you wouldn't need their services too much anymore. That's why it's far more lucrative to treat you and not cure you.

This is what I've learned in my 30+ years of treatment for my disabilities and pain. My disabilities were created by a car accident when a drunk driver ran a red light into the car I was riding in. My pain was created by my diet. It was this diet that I had been consuming for most of my life that was at the root of almost all of my pain. That's because I followed what the USDA recommended for our diet. The USDA recommends a diet based on what farmers can provide and not what is healthy to eat and this where the problem with America's pandemics of diabetes, heart disease, cancer and Alzheimer's disease come from.

What initially started out as a problem with glycation has turned into extreme glycation due to the amounts of glyphosate herbicide sprayed multiple times as ordered recommended by Monsanto for their farmers. As you just read above, they told to spray it just days before harvesting. This ensures that it gets into your food supply, regardless of what you eat, unless you're not eating the grains (cereal or legume). It's these foods that create a lions portion of the glycation, to begin with. Now, Monsanto wants to help that glycation along by forcing the enzyme inhibiting weed killer down your throats.

It's no wonder cancer, diabetes, dementia and all disease involved with inflammation have run rampant for the last 30 years. This also includes Parkinson's as displayed by this graph. This is a graph of the rise in Parkinson's deaths since the use of Roundup started over 40 years ago. Most of 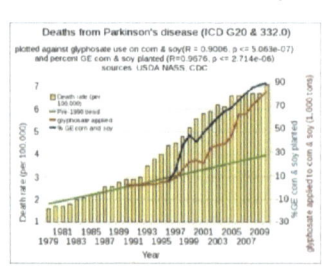 the increase has come in the last 20 years since the use of it has spread worldwide.

I hope it's easier to see now, how this industry does not have your best health in mind while growing the food you put on your table, for your family to eat. Now that you know what's at the root of all modern disease that has been plaguing the world ever since we've been eating grains, you also know that it's been amplified exponentially over the last 40 years. Grains which have always thought to be a healthy staple are inherently bad for us. Although they're able to sustain us, they're just as able to shorten our lives by the glycation that they create in the body. Now you know the missing link in this puzzle of why mankind has been plagued by these modern diseases ever since the start of civilization and why those diseases have been ramped up over the last 40 years, and really intensified in the last 20 years.

Monsanto denies this. They have to. Their business plan relies on the public not knowing this information. If the public knew that they were eating poisonous glyphosate herbicide every time they had a corn chip or bagel, or even just their oatmeal in the morning, how long do you think Monsanto's business would continue to thrive?

Here's your first clue to what this food does to you; my health since I quit eating it has improved so much that I experience very little pain now. I never take medication. I never get sick. I always have energy. From the time I get up in the morning (which is a little after sunup) until the time I go to bed (which is always 12 AM – 2 AM). I take very few breaks, if any, once I start working and I don't stop to eat. I pause to make a cup of Hot Chocolate around 8 or 8:30 PM, one of two or three that I'll drink before I go to bed, and then go right back to work, sipping my Hot Chocolate while I work.

Since I started my keto diet 3 years ago, I've lost my hunger cycle along with an expanded stomach that I had to keep full of carbs, just to keep my appetite under control. What I didn't know at that time was that my appetite was never under my control. It was always under the control of the industry that fed me. That's because I followed their advice. That advice that I followed was to make grains the largest part of my diet. So I ate grains every day, just like you're doing. But you still get sick, I don't. I won't get sick because I've broken the habit, the addiction that keeps you from kicking your habit.

This is a habit that's been imposed upon you and not by your choice, consciously. You were inflicted with this addiction when you were an infant and had no control over the food you ate. Too bad your mother didn't know then what she was doing to you, to guarantee your addiction. The food industry knew. That's why there's so much sugar in baby food, formula, and medicine. It's because it satiates so quickly it immediately calms a baby down. Whenever you can quiet a crying baby, it's assumed you're being a good mother. How many "good mothers" have addicted their kids by not knowing?

1. The dangers of sugar
2. The addictive nature of sugar
3. The glycative effects of sugar
4. The addition of Roundup to all sugar

Is this the kind of food you want your baby to eat? It's the kind of food you're eating. This is the kind of food that's giving you headaches and stomach aches. I know. I lived it for close to 60 years. It was imposed on me by my mother. She thought she was feeding me clean healthy food to grow on. It may have been food to grow on, but it wasn't healthy or clean. The clean food factor didn't come around until Monsanto invented their glyphosate herbicide, Roundup. After the emergence of Roundup on the market, modern diseases skyrocketed and have not slowed down since. The rate of these diseases will continue to increase until Roundup is no longer used. (What will happen to the millions of dollars invested in Monsanto when their products are deemed carcinogenic?)

This is why Monsanto can't afford this profitable, yet deadly behavior to discontinue. Their bottom line depends on this ruse continuing and continuing for as long as they can make money off of it. It depends on it, from two angles, from the crop seed side as well as the pharmaceutical side (even though they've supposedly divested themselves of their pharmaceutical holdings). I'm sure they all still have multiple stock options in both industries and if you think that won't influence their decisions, I think, you need to think again.

The use of Roundup is not going to wane as long as Monsanto is making millions of dollars on the sale of it. Over the last 20 years over 2.6 billion lbs of Roundup have been sprayed on U.S. farmland, according to **ECOWatch.com** With all that herbicide sprayed on your food, how much of do you think you could stay away from? If you eat food from a grocery store or a restaurant, you're eating Roundup with the food you eat. Monsanto makes certain of that. They have for the last 40 years. Are you starting to see the correlation of the addition of the herbicide and the condition of your health? Whatever glycation these grains create in the first place is magnified by the Roundup that's been sprayed on the crops these foods come from. Your addiction to these crops and their subsequent foods is what's behind the pandemics of cancer, diabetes, heart disease, hypertension, dementia (including Alzheimer's and Parkinson's diseases) and **all** other diseases involved with inflammation. Basically, that means that if you're eating these grains, both cereal and legume, you're subjecting your body to poisons that are not only carcinogenic, they're atherosclerotic and inflammatory, to say the least. If they are even close to being responsible for cancer, I'm not going to chance to eat them ever again. Now I'm really happy I quit and it explains why I've felt so good since I quit. It's easier to understand now why so many people are going ketogenic.

Remember when I **mentioned** that glyphosate is an enzyme inhibiting chemical that's an active ingredient in Roundup that it's also used as a component in many medicines to make the medicine more effective? This is the legal corporate engineering Monsanto has formulated over the last 30+ years, to take more and more of your money. And it's all for the sake of profits. Health? Well, that's just collateral damage.

Enzyme inhibitors are commonly used in medicine as well. The same enzyme inhibitors that are used in the roundup are also used in some heart medications. (I'll bet if the person knew that the food that this industry gave them to eat for the last 30 years, gave them that food to get them to buy their medicine years later, they would have made better choices when they had the option to.) I've got to hand it to Monsanto, though, in terms of business savvy. This is the ultimate ruse. It's a gargantuan ruse perpetrated on the public without anyone finding out until now.

Now I also know why so much drug use leads to more and more drug use. It's a true dependence inflicted upon you by Monsanto. First, they addict you to sugar. Then they addict you to the drugs you'll need to fight the pain created by the sugar. Then they'll addict you to a cycle of prescription medication that will continuously create a need for more medication until the cycle ends in premature death. The saddest part of this story is you'll probably never believe it...until you break your addiction. The next saddest part is that you were never told, until now.

The industry has formed its own "*Industry Task Force on Glyphosate*" to disseminate information on how healthy glyphosate is and how much benefit it is to the environment, yet more and more consumers are becoming aware of its inherent dangers. More and more people are waking up to the true poisoning that this enzyme inhibiting herbicide inflicts on the uneducated public.

Isn't it bad enough that the grains they grow glycate proteins and cholesterol? Do they really need to make it more poisonous? It's already at the heart of all major modern disease, isn't that enough? Are they really that greedy that they're willing to poison the whole world to increase their profits, even more? Wouldn't you consider this criminal?

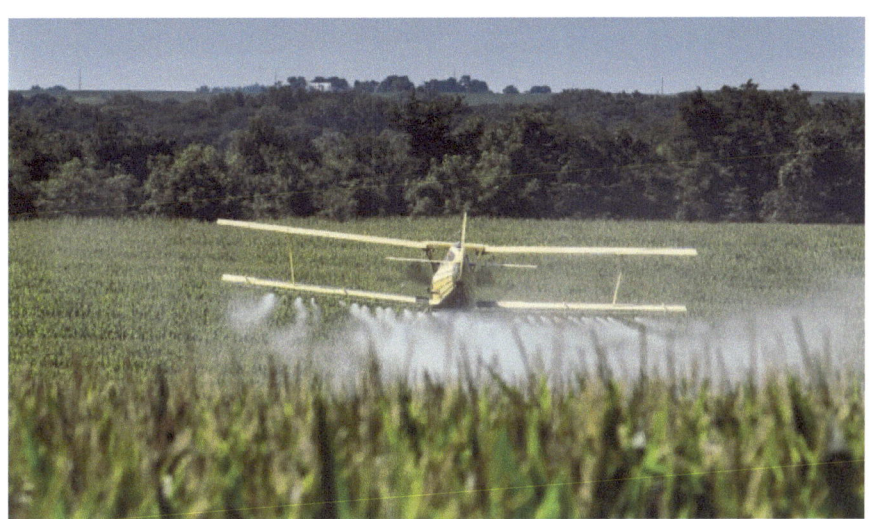

CHAPTER 3

THE GLYPHOSATE POISONING OF AMERICA

Monsanto's Covert Chemical Terrorism

Who knew that our greatest terrorist threat would be a clandestine threat from inside our country and it doesn't carry a gun or bomb, or any kind of explosives, for that fact. This threat is a completely hidden threat, making it the worst threat we've ever faced. This threat comes from your diet. It's been forced upon you since you were a baby. This threat comes right from the core of the glucose ruse. This threat **is** the glucose ruse.

It's in something you eat multiple times a day. In all actuality, your hunger cycle is the instrument of your destruction, with this threat. It's your hunger cycle that locks you into the cycle of destruction that glycation is responsible for, as its the glucose that's responsible for all inflammation, which in turn, is responsible for all modern disease. Since it's glucose that's at the heart of all glycation, that puts it at the heart of all inflammation, as well. Being at the heart of inflammation means it's at the heart of all modern disease.

This glycation gets compounded exponentially by an herbicide that gets sprayed on it as a crop, multiple times, as late as two weeks before it's harvested. The herbicide that's widest used in the industry, is glyphosate, patented in 1970 by Monsanto. They lost their patent in 2000, so the *Roundup* brand weed killer can now be sold under any name, making it the widest used herbicide ever. (2.6 billion lbs of glyphosate have been sprayed over the last 20 years.) All of that glyphosate was sprayed on what you eat, meaning if you bought your groceries at a grocery store or ate at a restaurant, you ingested a good portion of what was sprayed.

Glyphosate is an enzyme inhibitor. That's how it works. It works through senescence. Senescence is the science of aging, and that's how these enzyme inhibitors work. They age the weed so fast that it dies within three days. This may be great for the farmer and his crop, but it's having a disastrous effect on your health. This is due to all the glyphosate that's sprayed on these crops over their lifetime. The last time is to desiccate the crop two weeks before harvest. This is done so there's less green seed in the crop, for a better harvest. Green seed isn't good for grinding, as it's too wet.

No crop that I know of gets washed off before it goes to the mill for grinding. That means that you're eating what's just been sprayed on these crops every time you eat any grains that it's been sprayed on. (And it's sprayed on almost all grains. Monsanto is doing as much as they can to own every farmer in the country to distribute these GMO crop seeds too.) Monsanto seems to want to spread as much glyphosate around the world as they possibly can and it's not doing anybody's health any good. Increased rates of heart disease, cancer, and

Alzheimer's disease prove this. An increase of autism follows the same line on the same graph for the same amount of years. There is a correlation. Enzyme inhibiting is not conducive to good health. The two don't go together.

All this damage from the enzyme inhibitors in the glyphosate that's done to your hormones, when you eat this food, is no small matter. These hormones are important hormones affecting digestion, hunger, and sleep. (Those are the very same things affected by your diet, also.) Where's the similarity? It's explained in the way it affects its targeted enzymes, like tyrosine, tryptophan, and phenylalanine. These are all enzymes that influence your hunger, digestion and sleep hormones. If you have problems in any of these areas, this is your answer why.

It involves your consumption of glyphosate. (I'll bet you didn't know that, did you?) Would you eat it in the first place, if you knew? You probably would because you've been addicted to what they spray this substance on, without even knowing it. This was literally done right under your nose, when you were fed, as a baby. The industry makes certain that this substance gets into most all baby food. This ensures that you have no choice in this addiction. It ensures your lifetime of compliance in feeding the addiction. It also guarantees your compliance in the second half of the glucose ruse, the need for pharmaceuticals for the greatest portion of your life.

This is displayed in all these graphs below, as the increase of glyphosate usage mirrors the increase in disease. Are you one of these statistics? If you eat bread, I'm afraid you are.

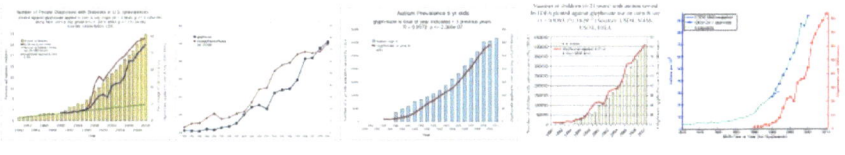

Targeted enzymes that influence the senescence of plants also influence the senescence of your body. They are important enzymes your body uses for digestion, sleep and controlling hunger;

Glyphosate is absorbed through foliage, and minimally through roots, and transported to growing points. It inhibits a plant enzyme involved in the synthesis of three aromatic amino acids: tyrosine, tryptophan, and phenylalanine. Therefore, it is effective only on actively growing plants and is not effective as a pre-emergence herbicide. An increasing number of crops have been genetically engineered to be tolerant of glyphosate (e.g. Roundup Ready soybean, the first Roundup Ready crop, also created by Monsanto) which allows farmers to use glyphosate as a post-emergence herbicide against weeds. The development of glyphosate resistance in weed species is emerging as a costly problem. While glyphosate and formulations such as Roundup have been approved by regulatory bodies worldwide, concerns about their effects on humans and the environment persist. Many

regulatory and scholarly reviews have evaluated the relative toxicity of glyphosate as an herbicide. The German Federal Institute for Risk Assessment toxicology review in 2013 found that "the available data is contradictory and far from being convincing" with regard to correlations between exposure to glyphosate formulations and risk of various cancers, including non-Hodgkin lymphoma (NHL). A meta-analysis published in 2014 identified an increased risk of NHL in workers exposed to glyphosate formulations. In March 2015 the World Health Organization's International Agency for Research on Cancer classified glyphosate as
"probably carcinogenic in humans" (category 2A) based on epidemiological studies, animal studies, and in vitro

- In November 2015, the European Food Safety Authority published an updated assessment report on glyphosate, concluding that "the substance is unlikely to be genotoxic (i.e. damaging to DNA) or to pose a carcinogenic threat to humans." Furthermore, the final report clarified that while other, probably carcinogenic, glyphosate-containing formulations may exist, studies "that look solely at the active substance glyphosate do not show this effect. In May 2016, the Joint FAO/WHO Meeting on Pesticide Residues concluded that "glyphosate is unlikely to pose a carcinogenic risk to humans from exposure through the diet", even at doses as high as 2,000 mg/kg body weight orally.

These targeted enzymes are important for digestion and hunger

- 1*Tyrosine* influences hunger by controlling enzymes that control how receptors react to stimuli that control your hunger. Tyrosine is a precursor to Dopamine, your primary hormone influencing hunger. This is the hormone triggered by leptin, your satiety hormone. If it takes more leptin to trigger the dopamine, it's going to take more food to trigger the leptin. Was this engineered intentionally?

- 2*Tryptophan* is also a precursor to serotonin and melatonin. Serotonin is another feel-good hormone that's affected by glyphosate. Melatonin is the hormone that allows you to sleep. without it, you're going to have trouble sleeping. Is it no wonder why so many people suffer from insomnia now? (They sell medicine for that, don't they?)

- 3*Phenylalanine* Phenylalanine is a precursor to tyrosine; the monoamine neurotransmitters dopamine, norepinephrine (noradrenaline), and epinephrine (adrenaline); and the skin pigment melanin. That was according to Wikipedia. All of those enzymes influence your hunger.

The WHO has finally recognized glyphosate as a **GROUP 2 CARCINOGEN**, meaning that it probably causes cancer. We know that it affects your sleep, hunger, and digestion, let's see if these chemicals can be responsible for cancer. The evidence for this lies in the multiple graphs showing the increase of glyphosate increasing right alongside the increase of multiple disorders and disease, including autism.

Monsanto's *Roundup* Ruse

In Monsanto's desire to spread as much of this on the earth as possible, they're poisoning every bit of food you eat, unless you grow your own and raise and butcher your own meat. All forage for feed is sprayed multiple times, maybe even more than the grain used for your bread. Cattle slaughtered for beef, never live long enough to get cancer, yet it goes into their food supply. 1,8 billion lbs in 20 years have been dumped on your food supplies. Ultimately, it goes into your body in multiple avenues, increasing the amount you consume, thereby increasing the number of enzyme inhibitors affecting your health. This has brought the pharmaceutical industry record profits, not to mention what it's brought Monsanto and their crop seed companies, pharmaceutical companies, and chemical wing of their manufacturing. Monsanto has engineered clandestine distemper on our health without us even knowing or approving of it.

It's not been good for the unsuspecting public who are still condemned to eating this food to feed their addiction as evidenced by these studies from PMC;

- ***Glyphosate, pathways to modern diseases III: Manganese, neurological diseases, and associated pathologies***

    Glyphosate is a likely cause of the recent epidemic of celiac disease. Glyphosate residues are found in wheat due to the increasingly widespread practice of staging and desiccation of wheat right before harvest. Many of the pathologies associated with celiac disease can be explained by disruption of CYP enzymes. Celiac patients have a shortened life span, mainly due to an increased risk to cancer, most especially non-Hodgkin's lymphoma, which has also been linked to glyphosate. Celiac disease trends over time match well with the increase in glyphosate usage on wheat crops.

    Glyphosate is also neurotoxic. Its mammalian metabolism yields two products: Aminomethylphosphonic acid (AMPA) and glyoxylate, with AMPA being at least as toxic as glyphosate. Glyoxylate is a highly reactive glycating agent, which will disrupt the function of multiple proteins in cells that are exposed. Glycation has been directly implicated in Parkinson's disease (PD). Glyphosate has been detected in the brains of malformed piglets. In a report produced by the Environmental Protection Agency (EPA), over 36% of 271 incidences involving acute glyphosate poisoning involved neurological symptoms, indicative of glyphosate toxicity in the brain and nervous system.

    In the remainder of this paper, we first introduce the link between glyphosate and manganese (Mn) dysbiosis and briefly describe the main biological roles of Mn. We then describe how glyphosate's disruption of gut bacteria may be a major player in the recent epidemic of antibiotic resistance. We then explain how glyphosate can influence the uptake of arsenic and aluminum, and propose similar mechanisms at work with Mn. In the next section, we describe how Mn deficiency can lead to a reduction in Lactobacillus in the gut, and we link this to anxiety disorder. We follow with a discussion on mitochondrial dysfunction associated with suppressed Mn superoxide dismutase (Mn-SOD), and then a section on implications of Mn deficiency for oxalate metabolism. The following section explains how Mn deficiency can lead to the overexpression of ammonia and glutamate in many neurological diseases. The next two sections show how Mn accumulation in the liver is linked to cholestasis and high serum low-density lipoprotein (LDL), and how this can also induce increased susceptibility to Salmonella poisoning. We then identify a role for Mn in chondroitin sulfate synthesis and the implications for osteomalacia. The next two sections explain how glyphosate exposure can lead to Mn toxicity in the brain, and discuss two neurological diseases that are associated with excess Mn, PD and prion diseases. After a section on the link between male infertility and Mn deficiency in the testes, we discuss evidence of exposure to glyphosate and end with a short summary of our findings.

The report goes on to detail how this herbicide is involved in suppressing dopamine which leads to an overactive thyroid. It's also involved in ;

1. **MICROBIAL ANTIBIOTIC INTOLERANCE**

    Manganese (Mn) is an often overlooked but important nutrient, required in small amounts for multiple essential functions in the body. A recent study on cows fed genetically modified Roundup®-Ready feed revealed a severe depletion of serum Mn. Glyphosate, the active ingredient in Roundup®, has also been shown to severely deplete Mn levels in plants. Here, we investigate the impact of Mn on physiology, and its association with gut dysbiosis as well as neuropathologies such as autism, Alzheimer's disease (AD), depression, anxiety syndrome, Parkinson's disease (PD), and prion diseases. Glutamate overexpression in the brain in association with autism, AD, and other neurological diseases can be explained by Mn deficiency. Mn superoxide dismutase protects mitochondria from oxidative damage, and mitochondrial dysfunction is a key feature of autism and Alzheimer's. Chondroitin sulfate synthesis depends on Mn, and its deficiency leads to osteoporosis and osteomalacia. Lactobacillus, depleted in autism, depend critically on Mn for antioxidant protection. Lactobacillus probiotics can treat anxiety, which is a comorbidity of autism and chronic fatigue syndrome. Reduced gut Lactobacillus leads to overgrowth of the pathogen, Salmonella, which is resistant to glyphosate toxicity, and Mn plays a role here as well. Sperm motility depends on Mn, and this may partially explain increased rates of infertility and birth defects. We further reason that, under conditions of adequate Mn in the diet, glyphosate, through its disruption of bile acid homeostasis, ironically promotes toxic accumulation of Mn in the brainstem, leading to conditions such as PD and prion diseases.

2. **MANGANESE DYSBIOSIS DUE TO GLYPHOSATE**

Remarkably, Mn deficiency can explain many of the pathologies associated with autism and Alzheimer's disease (AD). The incidence of both of these conditions has been increasing at an alarming rate in the past two decades, in step with the increased usage of glyphosate on corn and soy crops in the United States, as shown in Figures

3. ANALOGY WITH ARSENIC AND ALUMINUM

Chronic kidney disease is clearly associated with multiple environmental toxicants. There has been an epidemic in recent years in kidney failure among young agricultural workers in Central America, India, and Sri Lanka, particularly those working in the sugar cane fields. A recent paper reached the unmistakable conclusion that glyphosate plays a critical role in this epidemic. A growing practice of spraying sugar cane with glyphosate as a ripener and desiccant right before the harvest has led to much greater exposure to the workers in the fields. The authors, who focused their studies on affected workers in rice paddies in Sri Lanka, identified a synergistic effect of arsenic, which contaminated the soil in the affected regions. This paper is highly significant because it proposes a mechanism whereby glyphosate greatly increases the toxicity of arsenic through chelation, which promotes uptake by the gut. Glyphosate also depletes glutathione (GSH) and glutathione S transferase (GST) is a critical enzyme for liver detoxification of arsenic. As a consequence, excess arsenic in the kidney causes acute kidney failure, without evidence of other symptoms such as diabetes usually preceding kidney failure.

4. ANALOGY WITH ARSENIC AND ALUMINUM
5. MN-SUPEROXIDE DISMUTASE AND MITOCHONDRIAL DYSFUNCTION
6. GUT BACTERIA DYSBIOSIS AND ANXIETY
7. AMMONIA, GLUTAMATE, AND NEUROTOXICITY

In this section, we will show that both glutamate and ammonia are implicated as neurotoxins in connection with autism and other neurological diseases, and we will offer the simple explanation that Mn deficiency leads to impaired activity of glutamine synthase and arginase, both of which utilize Mn as a cofactor. Mn deficiency can also explain the increased risk of epilepsy found in autism, due to the fact that Mn decreases T2 relaxation time. Mn-deprived rats are more susceptible to convulsions.

Many diseases and conditions are currently on the rise in step with glyphosate usage in agriculture, particularly on GM crops of corn and soy. These include autism, AD, PD, anxiety disorder, osteoporosis, inflammatory bowel disease, renal lithiasis, osteomalacia, cholestasis, thyroid dysfunction, and infertility. All of these conditions can be substantially explained by the dysregulation of Mn utilization in the body due to glyphosate.

It may seem implausible that glyphosate could be toxic to humans, given the fact that government regulators appear nonchalant about steadily increasing residue limits, and that the levels in food and water are rarely monitored by government agencies, presumably due to lack of concern. However, a paper by Antoniou ET AL. provided a scathing indictment of the European regulatory process regarding glyphosate's toxicity, focusing on potential teratogenic effects. They identified several key factors leading to a tendency to overlook potential toxic effects. These include using animal studies that are too short or have too few animals to achieve statistical significance, disregarding IN VITRO studies or studies with exposures that are higher than what is expected to be realistically present in food, and discarding studies that examine the effects of glyphosate formulations rather than pure glyphosate, even though formulations are a more realistic model of the natural setting and are often orders of magnitude more toxic than the active ingredient in pesticides. Regulators also seemed unaware that chemicals that act as endocrine disruptors (such as glyphosate often have an inverted dose-response relationship, wherein very low doses can have more acute effects than higher doses. Teratogenic effects have been demonstrated in human cell lines. An IN VITRO study showed that glyphosate in parts per trillion can induce human breast cancer cell proliferation.

8. PARKINSON'S DISEASE
9. PRION DISEASES
10. OSTEOMALACIA AND ARTHRITIS

This is only a partial list of what this herbicide is responsible for. Visit the link at the head of this section for the full story. You should visit it, if only for your health's concern. This just points out the fact that what you eat has more impact on your health than anything else. It would be nice if you could get away from it, but you can't. The pollution is everywhere you go for food. You have to produce your own food to be completely free from this curse.

It's cursing you not only through the grains you eat but through the damage done to feed crops, contaminating beef, pork, chicken, turkey and even dairy cows, poisoning even the cheese, milk and butter you buy. The only way you can get around this ruse is to grow your own food and raise and butcher your own meat. Monsanto has every other path sewn up, tighter than a drum. To eat grains is to court death. It's become that simple. These reports from PubMed give you an idea of what over 150 other reports say;

- *Glyphosate, pathways to modern diseases II: Celiac sprue and gluten intolerance*

Celiac disease, and, more generally, gluten intolerance, is a growing problem worldwide, but especially in North America and Europe, where an estimated 5% of the population now suffers from it. Symptoms include nausea, diarrhea, skin rashes, macrocytic anemia, and depression. It is a multifactorial disease associated with numerous nutritional deficiencies as well as reproductive issues and increased risk to thyroid disease, kidney failure, and cancer. Here, we propose that glyphosate, the active ingredient in the herbicide, Roundup®, is the most important causal factor in this epidemic. Fish exposed to glyphosate develop digestive problems that are reminiscent of celiac disease. Celiac disease is associated with imbalances in gut bacteria that can be fully explained by the known effects of glyphosate on gut bacteria. Characteristics of celiac disease point to impairment in many cytochrome P450 enzymes, which are involved with detoxifying environmental toxins, activating vitamin D3, catabolizing vitamin A, and maintaining bile acid production and sulfate supplies to the gut. Glyphosate is known to inhibit cytochrome P450 enzymes. Deficiencies in iron, cobalt, molybdenum, copper and other rare metals associated with celiac disease can be attributed to glyphosate's strong ability to chelate these elements. Deficiencies in tryptophan, tyrosine, methionine, and selenomethionine associated with celiac disease match glyphosate's known depletion of these amino acids. Celiac disease patients have an increased risk of non-Hodgkin's lymphoma, which has also been implicated in glyphosate exposure. Reproductive issues associated with celiac diseases, such as infertility, miscarriages, and birth defects, can also be explained by glyphosate. Glyphosate residues in wheat and other crops are likely increasing recently due to the growing practice of crop desiccation just prior to the harvest. We argue that the practice of "ripening" sugar cane with glyphosate may explain the recent surge in kidney failure among agricultural workers in Central America. We conclude with a plea to governments to reconsider policies regarding the safety of glyphosate residues in foods.

- **GUT BACTERIA**

    We then show that glyphosate is associated with an overgrowth of pathogens along with an inflammatory bowel disease in animal models. A parallel exists with celiac disease where the bacteria that are positively and negatively affected by glyphosate are overgrown or underrepresented respectively in association with celiac disease in humans.

- **CYP ENZYME IMPAIRMENT AND SULFATE DEPLETION**
- **RETINOIC ACID, CELIAC DISEASE, AND REPRODUCTIVE ISSUES**
- **ANEMIA AND IRON**

    Glyphosate's chelating action can have profound effects on iron in plants. Glyphosate interferes with iron assimilation in both glyphosate-resistant and glyphosate-sensitive soybean crops. It is therefore conceivable that glyphosate's chelation of iron is responsible for the refractory iron deficiency present in celiac disease.

- **MOLYBDENUM DEFICIENCY**
- **SELENIUM AND THYROID DISORDERS**
- **INDOLE AND KIDNEY DISEASE**

- **NUTRITIONAL DEFICIENCIES**

    Glyphosate disrupts the synthesis of tryptophan and tyrosine in plants and in gut bacteria, due to its interference with the shikimate pathway, which is its main source of toxicity to plants. Glyphosate also depletes methionine in plants and microbes. A study on serum tryptophan levels in children with celiac disease revealed that untreated children had significantly lower ratios of tryptophan to large neutral amino acids in the blood, and treated children also had lower levels, but the imbalance was less severe.

- **Cancer**

    Chronic inflammation, such as occurs in celiac disease, is a major source of oxidative stress and is estimated to account for 1/3 of all cancer cases worldwide. Oxidative stress leads to DNA damage and increased risk of a genetic mutation. Several population-based studies do have confirmed that patients with celiac disease suffer from increased mortality, mainly due to malignancy. These include increased the risk to non-Hodgkin's lymphoma, adenocarcinoma of the small intestine, and squamous cell carcinomas of the esophagus, mouth, and pharynx, as well as melanoma. The non-Hodgkin's lymphoma was not restricted to gastrointestinal sites, and the increased risk remained following a gluten-free diet.

- **Proposed transglutaminase-glyphosate interactions**
- **Evidence of glyphosate exposure in humans and animals**
- **Kidney disease in agricultural workers**

In another study in the PMC database of over 164 studies done on this subject;

- **Republished study: long-term toxicity of a Roundup herbicide and a Roundup-tolerant genetically modified maize**

    Biochemical analyses confirmed very significant chronic kidney deficiencies, for all treatments and both sexes; 76% of the altered parameters were kidney-related. In treated males, liver congestions and necrosis were 2.5 to 5.5 times higher. Marked and severe nephropathies were also generally 1.3 to 2.3 times greater. In females, all treatment groups showed a two- to threefold increase in mortality, and deaths were earlier. This difference was also evident in three male groups fed with GM maize. All results were hormone- and sex-dependent, and the pathological profiles were comparable. Females developed large mammary tumors more frequently and before controls; the pituitary was the second most disabled organ; the sex hormonal balance was modified by consumption of GM maize and Roundup treatments. Males presented up to four times more large palpable tumors starting 600 days earlier than in the control group, in which only one tumor was noted. These results may be explained by not only the non-linear endocrine-

disrupting effects of Roundup but also by the overexpression of the EPSPS transgene or other mutational effects in the GM maize and their metabolic consequences.

Our findings show that the differences in multiple organ functional parameters seen from the consumption of NK603 GM maize for 90 days escalated over 2 years into severe organ damage in all types of test diets. This included the lowest dose of R administered (0.1 ppb, 50 ng/L G equivalent) of R formulation administered, which is well below permitted MRLs in both the USA (0.7 mg/L) and European Union (100 ng/L). Surprisingly, there was also a clear trend in increased tumor incidence, especially mammary tumors in female animals, in a number of the treatment groups. Our data highlight the inadequacy of 90-day feeding studies and the need to conduct long-term (2 years) investigations to evaluate the life-long impact of GM food consumption and exposure to complete pesticide formulations.

Tumors are reported in line with the requirements of OECD chronic toxicity protocols 452 and 453, which require all 'lesions' (which by definition include tumors) to be reported. These findings are summarized in Figure 4. The results are presented in the form of real-time cumulative curves (each step corresponds to an additional tumor in the group). Only the growing largest palpable growths (above a diameter of 17.5 mm in females and 20 mm in males) are presented (for example, see Figure 5A, B, C). These were found to be in 95% of cases non-regressive tumors (Figure 5D, E, F, G, H, I, J) and were not infectious nodules. These arose from time to time; then, most often disappeared and were not different from controls after bacterial analyses. The real tumors were recorded independently of their grade, but dependent on their morbidity, since non-cancerous tumors can be more lethal than those of cancerous nature, due to internal hemorrhaging or compression and obstruction of the function of vital organs, or toxins or hormone secretions. These tumors progressively increased in size and number, but not proportionally to the treatment dose, over the course of the experiment (Figure 4). As in the case of rates of mortality (Figure 6), this suggests that a threshold in effect was reached at the lower doses. Tumor numbers were rarely equal but almost always more than in controls for all treated groups, often with a two- to threefold increase for both sexes. Tumors began to reach a large size on average 94 days before controls in treated females and up to 600 days earlier in two male groups fed with GM maize (11 and 22% with or without R).

- **Glyphosate formulations induce apoptosis and necrosis in human umbilical, embryonic, and placental cells.**

We have evaluated the toxicity of four glyphosates (G)-based herbicides in Roundup formulations, from 10(5) times dilutions, on three different human cell types. This dilution level is far below agricultural recommendations and corresponds to low levels of residues in food or feed. The formulations have been compared to G alone and with its main metabolite AMPA or with one known adjuvant of R formulations,

> POEA. HUVEC primary neonate umbilical cord vein cells have been tested with 293 embryonic kidney and JEG3 placental cell lines. All R formulations cause total cell death within 24 h, through an inhibition of the mitochondrial succinate dehydrogenase activity, and necrosis, by the release of cytosolic adenylate kinase measuring membrane damage. They also induce apoptosis via activation of enzymatic caspases 3/7 activity. This is confirmed by characteristic DNA fragmentation, nuclear shrinkage (pyknosis), and nuclear fragmentation (karyorrhexis), which is demonstrated by DAPI in apoptotic round cells. G provokes only apoptosis, and HUVEC is 100 times more sensitive overall at this level. The deleterious effects are not proportional to G concentrations but rather depend on the nature of the adjuvants. AMPA and POEA separately and synergistically damage cell membranes like R but at different concentrations. Their mixtures are generally even more harmful to G. In conclusion, the R adjuvants like POEA change human cell permeability and amplify toxicity induced already by G, through apoptosis and necrosis. The real threshold of G toxicity must take into account the presence of adjuvants but also G metabolism and time-amplified effects or bioaccumulation. This should be discussed when analyzing the in vivo toxic actions of R. This work clearly confirms that the adjuvants in Roundup formulations are not inert. Moreover, the proprietary mixtures available on the market could cause cell damage and even death around residual levels to be expected, especially in food and feed derived from R formulation-treated crops.

This poses a major question in my mind; can the target in this ruse, be you and your money? It's obviously what the end result is and that's displayed in the record profits of the pharmaceutical industry. The more disease caused by this herbicide, the more medicine the pharmaceutical industry sells. Monsanto owns the crop seed companies. They own the chemical company that produces the herbicide, and they used to own the pharmaceutical corporations, so they're profiting much more than two or three times in this ruse. It's that simple. They're making money off of your ignorance of the facts. They've withheld information that's vital to your health. They've outright lied to you to keep you in the dark. They don't want you to know this information.

Only you can control this transformation of your health, this travesty of justice. Only you can say no to the grains that this herbicide poisons. It's your choice to remain a slave to Monsanto or be free. All you have to do is to give up the grains.

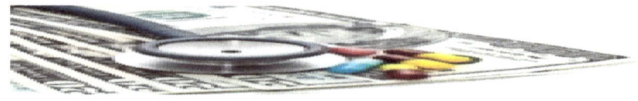

PART II

WHAT WERE DIRTY CARBS

ARE NOW POLLUTED CARBS

TOO MUCH SUGAR

- cardiovascular disease
- metabolic syndrome
- tooth decay
- hypoglycemia
- dizziness
- obesity
- allergies
- ADD/ADHD
- cholesterol
- type 2 diabetes
- hypertension
- colon & pancreatic cancer

CHAPTER 4
CALORIES, DO YOU WORRY ABOUT THEM?

Calories, do you worry about how many you eat? If you do, you're not alone. A lot of people do the very same thing, they count their calories. If you're one of those who does, I have a suggestion for you. To help make your job easier and you healthier; you shouldn't worry about how many calories you eat, as much as you should worry about where the calories come from.

Calories are essential to survive, so they're absolutely necessary and yes if you eat more, you weigh more. If you eat less, of course, you weigh less. That does make eating fewer calories crucial yet eating less to control them can be very difficult at the least if you're on a carb diet. The simple reason to this is because carbs make you hungry. They create and maintain a hunger cycle that you have no control over, without removing them. That makes, where you get your calories from, more important than how many you eat.

Are the calories you get from the food you eat most, from carbohydrates or are the calories from protein and fat? If you're eating calories from carbohydrates, under the guise of **healthy energy**, you're allowing those carbs to make the fat that your body needs to use for that energy. If you're getting your calories from fat and protein, you're feeding your body exactly what it needs to survive and thrive. Eating fats and protein also allows your body to heal itself from virtually anything. It is very little our bodies cannot heal from, as long as they don't have the influence of the glycation that's the result of carbohydrates contaminating their systems. That means if your body needs glucose, let it make its own.

Whatever glucose you can get from carbs, your body can supply, on its own. When your brain (which is the only part of your body that needs glucose) needs glucose, it can supply the brain with all it needs through a process of gluconeogenesis. Your body reformulates the glycogen in your body to pull glycose out of it to use whenever the brain needs the glucose. (Remember, glycose used to be the name for glucose.)The interesting thing about this little-known fact is that your body makes this glucose, regardless of how much you already have in your body from the carbs you eat.

This all points to the fact that your body will make the nutrients it needs, provided you feed it the proper foods, to begin with, and carbs are not in that group. Carbs make your body make its own fat. It makes that fat out of the carbs you eat with the hormone insulin. (That's an enzyme you don't want to be inhibited.) A healthier way to live is to allow your body to make its own glucose instead of fat. This does wonder for the body. As long as you eat enough protein to compensate for the loss of muscle tissue from gluconeogenesis, you'll never lose vital muscle tissue.

This is why long fasts help you cure most diseases. After your body uses up its own fat to fuel your body, it resets your body to produce growth hormones that not only help keep you thinner; they keep you healthier by repairing your systems for you (usually without the need for medication).

It does this by changing your hormones. The way in which many hormones work is affected by eliminating carbs from the diet. Insulin is soon replaced by glucagon which regulates the gluconeogenesis that takes place in your body whenever it needs glucose. This hormone regulates how fat is burned in your body, whereas insulin controls how fat is stored in your body. As long as you're eating carbs you're creating insulin and it's instructing all the fat you're making to be stored, instead of to be used.

When you remove the carbs from your diet; your body changes, from increasing its production of insulin to increasing the production of glucagon which in turn ramps up the burning of your fat. This is why keto diets work so good. It's also why carb diets work so bad. In short, carb diets add fat to your body to be stored, keto diets take fat from your body to be burned. Which sounds healthier to you?

DIRTY FOOD GIVES YOU DIRTY FUEL

That means when you continue a diet of carbs, you're forcing your body to make its own fat out of those carbs and this is where your problem lies. The fat your body turns the glucose into is not a clean burning fat. It's a dirty fat at best. It leaves glycated residue wherever it's burned. That, in turn, gums up your cells...all of them, including your brain cells, your heart cells, your kidney cells, liver cells, every cell that blood flows through including the blood vessels they flow through. This is the true danger in carbohydrate consumption. This danger has been magnified by the glyphosate herbicide Roundup, with its enzyme inhibiting chemicals.

Some of the enzymes that get affected are enzymes that influence behavior. Some of these behavioral enzymes influence your appetite, as well as digestion, making this enzyme inhibitor responsible for more of your hunger and less of your nutrition. (It could actually detract from your nutrition.)

POLLUTED FUEL COSTS YOU, YOUR LIFE

Could that be why Monsanto is so adamant about their product being safe? They must know, if they reduce the use of their enzyme inhibitors on crops they're going to cut down on the need for their medications, to counteract the changes those enzyme inhibitors impose on the body. and this could spell doom for their pharmaceutical industry.

If news like that were to leak out to the world, what would happen to the profits of the food producers that depend on the grain industry to provide them with their flour? What do you think that would to the profits of the pharmaceutical corporations Monsanto used to own? Don't you think that would have a major influence on them if everyone knew that it was actually all of the grain products that Monsanto is responsible for that is making them need the very medications that Monsanto's old pharmaceutical companies make?

I'm sure the pharmaceutical companies are still customers of Monsanto chemical division now, buying the same enzyme inhibitors to use in heart medication as well as many cancer medications. This practice leads only to more and more drug need by their consumers and this is how you get hooked. If you eat grains in any form you're one of their consumers.

This is what killed my mother and continues to kill over 20,000 mothers every day. This vicious cycle is courtesy of Monsanto's crop seed companies, Monsanto's herbicide companies through the production and spraying of Roundup, and what used to be Monsanto's corporate partner, Pharmacia. (Don't forget, they patented Celebrex 24 years ago.) Although I can understand if you did forget and why you forgot, it's in the food you eat. Now, can you see the danger?

Cutting down on the use of these herbicides will also cut down on the need to use these same chemicals to make the pharmaceuticals that help to counteract the damage done in the first place. This is the doom they've condemned our society to, an addiction that feeds itself into a pharmaceutical dependence. Their greed is more important to them than the health and safety of all America (and the world, for that fact). Their glyphosate ensures this for Monsanto even after their patent expired. It also ensures that America is not free, but still under the control of this industry and Monsanto.

*ACCORDING TO WIKIPEDIA; Glyphosate kills plants by interfering with the synthesis of the **aromatic** amino acids **phenylalanine**, **tyrosine**, and **tryptophan**. It does this by inhibiting the enzyme **5-enolpyruvylshikimate-3-phosphate synthase** (EPSPS), which **catalyzes** the reaction of **shikimate**-3-phosphate (S3P) and **phosphoenolpyruvate** to form 5-enolpyruvyl-shikimate-3-phosphate (EPSP). Glyphosate is absorbed through foliage and minimally through roots, meaning that it is only effective on actively growing plants and cannot prevent seeds from germinating. After* application, glyphosate is readily transported around the plant to grow roots and leaves and this **systemic** activity is important for its effectiveness. Inhibiting the enzyme causes shikimate to accumulate in plant tissues and diverts energy and resources away from other processes. While growth stops within hours of application, it takes several days for the leaves to begin **turning yellow**.

This is the damage it does to weeds but it can do the same kind of damage to your body by affecting the way your enzymes work. This makes your body waste a lot more energy, converting those glyphosated carbs into fat, so it can use them.

If you feed your body fat in the first place, you don't need to convert anything as the fat is "ready to use". This last little factor is what's important to know because it doesn't require your body to make fat out of the sugar. This is what drains your pancreas from its supply of insulin. It also glycates your blood and it's this glycation, that leads to more modern disease than any other one thing. If you can control glycation, you control all inflammation. Controlling all inflammation means that you're controlling all modern diseases created by inflammation.

This fact combined with the fact that Roundup affects the enzymes **phenylalanine**, **tyrosine**, and **tryptophan**, means that they're also affecting your hunger patterns, digestion, and sleep. That creates a double dipper for the food industry and pharmaceutical industry. And they do this legally, thanks to a patent law from 1954 and a ruling from an old Monsanto lawyer saying that modifying seeds for any purpose, is legal. I'm sure they didn't realize the consequences at the time their actions would have on humanity.

One of the enzymes affected in your body is Phenylalanine, a precursor for **tyrosine**; *the* **monoamine** *neurotransmitters* **dopamine**, **norepinephrine** *(noradrenaline), and* **epinephrine** *(adrenaline); and the skin* **pigment melanin**.

Affecting the phenylalanine is going to affect how your other hormones work that is influenced by these enzymes. Tryptophan is an enzyme that influences your hunger by influencing enzymes that affect hormones that are influenced by what you eat. This is why your hunger is greater now than it ever was in the past and this is why the obesity epidemic, diabetes epidemic, CVD epidemic, cancer epidemic and dementia epidemics have worsened alongside the increase of glyphosate sprayed on American crops.

That means you must get your calories from healthier sources like fats and protein. These are the foods your body prefers. It can live on carbs but carbs are only supposed to be used in times when we can't get the protein or fat and that's what makes cholesterol so important. Your LDL cholesterol is vital to your survival. If you accumulated this LDL from eating carbs, it's dirty LDL, which is going to leave a residue inside your cells and this is what turns carbs into poison. That residue is what leads to all the modern diseases known to man. If you can cut down on the residue, you control all disease.

Protein and fat have been the basis of our diet as far back as our species dates. We're not going to change that overnight by converting to a diet of carbs. That's insanity in my opinion. Homo Sapiens went through well over 100,000 years evolving from eating protein and fat, supplementing it with carbs to gradually eating more complex carb such as root vegetables and truly whole grains, as they picked them directly off the stalk and ate them. (This is the only way to get whole grains from these grasses.)

Today, the basis of our diet is carbs and we supplement it with protein and fat. This practice urged on by a grain industry that's interested only in profits and not public health, has proven deadly for all Americans. Since the expansion of the use of Roundup, this practice has become the deadliest practice that anyone can take part in. (Not even the extensive exercise our ancestors had from running all the time could have saved them from the ravages of this weed killer.)

This weed killer has turned into a people killer, through its enzyme inhibiting functions and this is something Monsanto continues to deny. (They've made lying to the public legal, with their placements in the USDA, FDA, EPA and probably the CDC all to ensure their success in carrying out this grandiose ruse that grains are healthy to eat and that you need to eat more of them. Hold on to that thought because we're going to look into why they're pushing this on the public like they are.

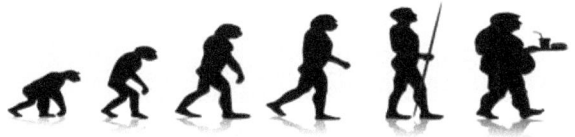

Thousands of years ago in our Paleolithic state, we were primarily carnivores. Although we did eat some leafs and tubers, we primarily ate protein and fat in all the game we ate. Our species took close to 90,000

years to cultivate wheat, which we've been eating as a major part of our diet, instead of a minor part, as it had been for those 90,000 years.

This cultivation of wheat was the beginning of modern diseases showing up in our bones after our death. As our consumption grew, so grew the frequency of occurrence and severity of the disease. This is simply the nature of grain food which is ultimately glycating food. Its speed of glycation has grown over the years to the point it's at now, exponentially more than it was just 100 years ago.

This is an inherent problem with carbs, especially this starchy type of carb, grains. Eating carbohydrates have its bad side, and it's called glycation. Protein can't create glycation. Fat can't create glycation. They both need the glucose to do that. That makes glucose a natural toxin that we've been eating for over 10,000 years, only to be ramped up in the last 50 years or so to where the proliferation of its use is now sending hoards of people to their premature deaths. It's also making these same people very sick for extended periods of time before they die. It also makes people sick while they continue to eat, what now are really dirty carbs, due to the glyphosate herbicide sprayed on them as many as four times before they reach your table. Think about that for a minute.

The bread you make your sandwich with is toxic. It's been poisoned right under your nose without your consent, or knowledge, which forces you to need the pharmaceuticals that this same company produces. Who knew that this addiction that's been forced upon you would claim your health with every bite you take?

You should know what addiction this is by now and what you can do about it. What they're selling as safe has escalated death rates from diabetes to brain cancer, from Alzheimer's to atherosclerosis, all evidenced by the rise in cancer rates in the farmers that work with this weed killer.

It's also evidenced by the rise in autism since the start of spraying, 40 years ago. Autism rates climbed steadily for 15 – 20 years from the early 70's when they started using glyphosate, until they too, skyrocketed in the 90's when glyphosate usage multiplied. Now glyphosate is at an all-time high with every rate of modern disease at an all-time high as well.

Yet Monsanto and its industry refuse to acknowledge the true damage they're doing to our society. It's their greed that's driving every pandemic known to modern man. From destroying our health to destroying the environment, Monsanto is leaving quite possibly the largest footprint on our ecosystem, medical system, the pharmaceutical system as well as our agricultural systems and legal/political systems. They've mastered the industrial destruction of mankind and they've done it well from an investor's view. I just wish it could be that well from a consumer's viewpoint.

They have orchestrated legal covert terrorism on an unsuspecting public, by saturating our diets with toxic food, without telling us. What they should have shared with us, was that they were using us as guinea pigs, for their experiment on the impact glyphosate has, on human physiology.

Their experiment has been disastrous for the American people, as well as the world, as glyphosate is breaking records in sales every year, especially since the patent expired 16 years ago. But this isn't supposed to be about glyphosate. This is about the calories you eat and where you get them from. The glyphosate sprayed grains just tells you, not to get your calories from that source as that source is now tainted, severely.

Do you get your calories from a dirty source like carbs or do you get them from efficient foods like protein and fats? Remember where I said that a gram of sugar has 4 calories and that a gram of fat has 9 calories? That only points to the fact that fat is 225% more efficient as a food source. (This is something Monsanto has lied to you, for about 30 years.) With fat being that much more efficient than sugar, it's no wonder that it's that much healthier.

Eating the proper fats feeds your body exactly what it's been running on ever since we've been running as a species. A run we did in our Paleolithic years. We ran all day long, either hunting food, tracking down food, or just running down our food. The funny thing about this is, they were all running on empty stomachs, all day long, and not running out of energy. They could only do this by not eating many carbs. Their bodies had to run on ketones and fat, ramped up by adiponectin and other hormones in their bodies that set their brains to grow. (Many Paleolithic species had larger craniums and brains then we currently do. This is due to their low carb diet and its influence on their growth hormones. Fasting does this also.) The ketogenic diet they were on also does this.

It was this constant practice of exercising every day that made their bodies produce the hormones that allowed them to advance faster than the other species. It was our ability to sweat and cool our bodies that allowed our ancestors to run down their game to feed their families. It was this kind of diet that our bodies ate for 10's of 1,000's for years. Not until the last 60 years or so did we become sedentary and start eating more of what used to take us a half a day of gathering to eat. Most people now get their calories without the gathering or the hunting or the running so they never burn up those calories. They store them. This is the nature of a carbohydrate diet. The same hormone (insulin) instructs the fat it just made to store itself as visceral fat around your midsection until you need it. Your problem is, you seldom need it so it stays as fat.

The bad thing about that is that this fat you just made out of your carbs is going to demand more fat to join it. Fat in your body shuts down the action of leptin, the satiety hormone. When this hormone isn't working right to tell you when to put down your spoon, it's demanding that your body consume more carbs to satisfy it. This leptin resistance leads directly to you needing to eat more and more, just to produce enough leptin to satisfy your addiction. And this is precisely why you should get your calories from protein and a much more efficient fat, rather than carbs. This is a metabolic syndrome, a precursor to diabetes. This is why the keto diet is taking off so much. It's not only a fat burning diet, it's a brain growing, muscle growing diet that truly gives you the best body and brain you can have.

You're probably asking, what kind of fat is good to eat? I've always been told that fat is bad. Until I learned that it isn't at all. It's healthy. Actually, it's very healthy. The industry that told you it was bad had an interest in selling you that idea so you would eat more carbs. They even recommended for you to eat them over the fat. That's because the grain industry is behind the recommendations for what you eat and they're interested is in supplying more grains for you to consume.

The healthiest fats to partake of are MCT fats, Medium Chain Triglycerides. They'll balance your cholesterol which is much healthier than just lowering it. Balancing it will actually lower your LDL by increasing your HDL. It's the HDL that cleans out your cells of the spent LDL that's been fed into them. If your body can't clean out the burned LDL out of your cells, the LDL backs up in your blood increasing your overall cholesterol. What could be worse?

Later they found out that a diet of fat won't lead you to any drug use. That's reserved for the carb diet and that may have been why this industry dissuaded everyone from consuming a diet of fat. Just like the sugar industry the grain industry has been lying to the public for greater than 60 years about the safety of their food. Now, they've amplified its danger by dousing it with more and more glyphosate right up until three days before harvest. How safe do you really think that makes the food you eat?

Remember the thought I asked you to hold on to earlier in this article, why Monsanto has been pushing the idea that grains are healthy to eat? The answer to that question is because this is a crop that can be marketed to farmers as making them more money by producing more crop. Yet they need to spread more Roundup, to do this, according to

Monsanto. (This is something many farmers don't agree with and are actively trying to resist. Monsanto's push to own every farmer on North American soil has taken many of these farmers to court where Monsanto has tied them up for years at a time, often, to get them to use their own GMO seed.)

This includes Canada where a majority of canola comes from, which happens to come from another Monsanto glyphosated crop. This is another one that they like to spray with Roundup right before harvesting to save the lower oil pods that drop off the crop and shatter losing much of the valuable canola oil. For the farmer, it's Roundup to the rescue. For the consumer, it's Roundup to the dinner table where it can continue its enzyme inhibiting actions in the bodies of your family.

Right after Monsanto patented their first seed in 1980, they purchased GD Searle chemicals, makes NutraSweet in 1985. This was about 14 years after they patented Roundup. Their Roundup has done a bang-up job of bringing the senescence of glyphosate to humans. Roundup is advertised as working through senescence, on how it kills weeds. That senescence is rubbing off on our population. It was 7 years after they patented seeds that they patented Celebrex setting themselves up to be a provider of foods that require an early departure to drugs and a never-ending cycle that never lets up until a premature death. (This makes me think, they'd patent the glycation of America if they could.) This current cycle of disease, disorder, and death goes back to 1954 and the plant act. That's when they made it legal to patent seeds, later leading to genetic modifying of crop seed, later leading to genetically modifying crop seed to survive multiple uses of an enzyme inhibiting herbicide that induces senescence in humans. This is the genetic modifying of humans by modifying their food. This food that gets modified just happens to be an addictive food that's been made more addictive by its modifying. If this isn't criminal, I don't know what is.

To prevent your premature death, look to make fat and protein the core of your diet. You don't have to eat nearly as much, or as often, as it's that dreaded hunger cycle that never appears in the keto diet. That's because of the arguably worst manifestation of a carbohydrate diet is the hunger cycle that's tied to it. I don't know anyone who would agree to that kind of forced behavior. Especially when that hunger gets magnified by what's been sprayed on it multiple times. It's clear to me that the more glyphosate that Monsanto sells, the more disease the public is going to fight. From autism to Alzheimer's, all modern diseases have increased right alongside the increase of glyphosate usage. The only blessing here is that we don't have to eat it. We can say no to glyphosate by not eating any grains, including sugar.

Chapter 5
Can Your Cancer be Cured or Just Treated?

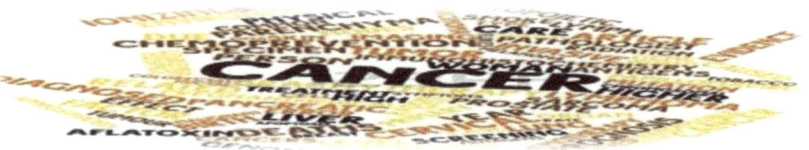

It's become evident to me that this problem of glycation goes much further than I previously thought when writing my second book, so it's important that I need to display a different chapter for the different types of damage that glycation induces. I'll list as many different types of cancer, here. All reports Of CVDs and other heart disorders will be located on the Atherosclerosis page. Dementias will 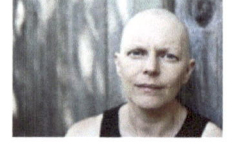 be on a separate page as well, with all other diseases and disorders inflammation is responsible for. The third bout of breast cancer was what took my mother.

Listed below from PubMed or PMC or the FDA are reports of studies done on the effects of glycation and its influence in any cancer, which is a direct result of glycation.

This report is dated Aug 9, 2016, and details AGEs role in lung cancer;

- *Advanced Glycation End-Products Enhance Lung Cancer Cell Invasion and Migration.*

Abstract

Effects of carboxymethyl-lysine (CML) and pentosidine, two advanced glycation end-products (AGEs), upon invasion and migration in A549 and Calu-6 cells, two non-small cell lung cancer (NSCLC) cell lines were examined. CML or pentosidine at 1, 2, 4, 8 or 16 μmol/L were added into cells. Proliferation, invasion, and migration were measured. CML or pentosidine at 4-16 μmol/L promoted invasion and migration in both cell lines and increased the production of reactive oxygen species, tumor necrosis factor-α, interleukin-6 and transforming growth factor-β1. CML or pentosidine at 2-16 μmol/L up-regulated the protein expression of AGE receptor, p47(phox), intercellular adhesion molecule-1 and fibronectin in test NSCLC cells. Matrix metalloproteinase-2 protein expression in A549 and Calu-6 cells was increased by CML or pentosidine at 4-16 μmol/L. These two AGEs at 2-16 μmol/L enhanced nuclear factor κ-B (NF-κ B) p65 protein expression and p38 phosphorylation in A549 cells. However, CML or pentosidine at 4-16 μmol/L up-regulated NF-κB p65 and p-p38 protein expression in Calu-6 cells. These findings suggest that CML and pentosidine, by promoting the invasion, migration, and production of associated factors, benefit NSCLC metastasis.

KEYWORDS: CML; invasion; migration; non-small cell lung cancer; pentosidine

I ran across this study on Polycystic Ovary Syndrome (PCOS). It details the influence that AGEs have on PCOS and how they contribute to the chronic inflammation and increased oxidative stress that is behind the disorder;

- ***Do Advanced Glycation End Products (AGEs) Contribute to the comorbidities of Polycystic Ovary Syndrome (PCOS)?***

Advanced glycation end products (AGEs) are formed both during the endogenous and exogenous reactions and are implicated in the process of aging, pathogenesis of diabetes, atherosclerosis, female fertility, and cancers. Food and smoking are the most important sources of exogenous AGEs in daily life. The biochemical composition of the meal, cooking methods, time and temperature of food preparation may impact AGEs formation, therefore Western-type diet, rich in animal-derived products as well as in fast foods seems to be the main source of AGEs. Both, endogenous and exogenous AGEs can act intracellularly or during serum interaction with cell surface receptors called RAGE influencing a variety of molecular pathways. Polycystic ovary syndrome (PCOS) is the most common endocrinopathy in women of reproductive age. The etiology of this disorder remains unclear, however, the environmental and genetic factors may play an important role in its pathogenesis. Nevertheless, PCOS women have increased factors for reproductive and cardiometabolic comorbidities. AGEs can contribute to the pathogenesis of PCOS as well as its consequences. It has been shown that chronic inflammation and increased oxidative stress may be a link between the mechanisms of AGEs action and the metabolic and reproductive consequences of PCOS. This review highlights that high dietary AGEs intake promotes deteriorating biological effects in women with PCOS, whereas AGEs restriction seems to have a beneficial impact on women health. Better understanding AGEs formation and biochemistry as well as AGE-mediated pathophysiological mechanisms may open new therapeutic avenues converging to the achievement of the complete treatment of PCOS and its consequences.

This appears to be indicative of glucose's influence in ovarian cancer. Is this something you thought you were eating when you had your English muffin this morning?

The following report submitted Sept 1, 2008, was concerned about RAGEs correlation with cervical cancer;

- ***Induction of receptor for advanced glycation end products by EBV latent membrane protein 1 and its correlation with angiogenesis and cervical lymph node metastasis in nasopharyngeal carcinoma.***

Abstract

PURPOSE:

The EBV oncoprotein, latent membrane protein 1 (LMP1), contributes to the metastasis of nasopharyngeal carcinoma (NPC) by inducing factors to promote tumor invasion and angiogenesis. The receptor for advanced glycation end products (RAGE) is associated with abnormal angiogenesis in diabetic microangiopathies. Moreover, some papers have suggested the association of RAGE overexpression with tumor metastasis; thus, the associations of RAGE with LMP1 and angiogenesis in NPC were examined.

EXPERIMENTAL DESIGN:

Forty-two patients with NPC were evaluated for expressions of LMP1, RAGE, and S100 proteins and for microvessel counts by immunohistochemistry. Then, the RAGE induction by LMP1 was examined with Western blotting and luciferase reporter assay.

RESULTS:

The microvessel counts were significantly higher in patients with high LMP1 expression or high RAGE expression compared with cases with low expressions (P=0.0049 and P<0.0001), respectively. Patients with advanced N classification were also significantly increased in these groups (P=0.0484 and P=0.0005). The expressions of LMP1 and RAGE proteins were clearly correlated in NPC tissues (P=0.0093). Transient transfection with an LMP1 expression plasmid induced RAGE protein in Ad-AH cells. The expression of LMP1 transactivated the RAGE promoter as shown by luciferase reporter assay. Mutation of the reporter at the nuclear factor-kappaB binding site (-671 to -663) abolished transactivation of the RAGE promoter by LMP1.

CONCLUSION:

These results suggest that LMP1-induced RAGE enhances lymph node metastasis through the induction of angiogenesis in NPC. The nuclear factor-kappaB binding site (-671 to -663) is essential for transactivation of the RAGE promoter by LMP1.

As of today January 10, 2017, this news still has not been spoken about in the media yet! No warnings about what causes glycation, only warnings against what doesn't cause it. That makes me wonder, is someone trying to hide this cure?

If that wasn't enough, another report that brain cancer is affected by glycation from 9 years ago, this is clear evidence in the following report, dated Mar 2008;

- **HMGB1 as an autocrine stimulus in human T98G glioblastoma cells: role in cell growth and migration.**

Abstract

HMGB1 (high mobility group box 1 protein) is a nuclear protein that can also act as an extracellular trigger of inflammation, proliferation, and migration, mainly through RAGE (the receptor for advanced glycation end products); HMGB1-RAGE interactions have been found to be important in a number of cancers. We investigated whether HMGB1 is an autocrine factor in human glioma cells. Western blots showed HMGB1 and RAGE expression in human malignant glioma cell lines. HMGB1 induced a dose-dependent increase in cell proliferation, which was found to be RAGE-mediated and involved the MAPK/ERK pathway. Moreover, in a wounding model, it induced a significant increase in cell migration, and RAGE-dependent activation of Rac1 was crucial in giving the tumor cells a motile phenotype. The fact that blocking DNA replication with anti-mitotic agents did not reduce the distance migrated suggests the independence of the proliferative and migratory effects. We also found that glioma cells contain HMGB1 predominantly in the nucleus, and cannot secrete it constitutively or upon stimulation; however, necrotic glioma cells can release HMGB1 after it has translocated from the nucleus to cytosol. These findings provide the first evidence supporting the existence of HMGB1/RAGE signaling pathways in human glioblastoma cells and suggest that HMGB1 may play an important role in the relationship between necrosis and malignancy in glioma tumors by acting as an autocrine factor that is capable of promoting the growth and migration of tumor cells.*

If that was 9 years ago, it was known then that even brain cancer is susceptible to glycation and its destructive effects. Why was this information withheld from the consumer know? Glycation seems to be at the root of all cancers. I can't seem to find cancer that isn't affected by glycation.

The following study was done in Sep 2013, and was concerned with the role of insulin and Insulin Growth Factor (IGF-1) signaling in cancer;

- **The key role of growth hormone — insulin — IGF-1 signaling in aging and cancer**

Abstract

Studies in mammals have led to the suggestion that hyperglycemia and hyperinsulinemia are important factors in aging. GH/Insulin/insulin-like growth factor 1 (IGF-1) signaling molecules that have been linked to longevity include daf-2 and INR and their homologs in mammals, and inactivation of the corresponding genes increases lifespan in nematodes, fruit flies, and mice. The life-prolonging effects of caloric restriction are likely related to decreasing IGF-1 levels. Evidence has emerged that antidiabetic drugs are promising candidates for both lifespan extension and prevention of cancer. Thus, antidiabetic drugs postpone spontaneous carcinogenesis in mice and rats, as well as chemical and radiation carcinogenesis in mice, rats, and hamsters. Furthermore, metformin seems to decrease the risk for cancer in diabetic patients...

Research conducted during the last 15-20 years firmly established insulin, insulin-like and homologous signaling as key regulators of aging and longevity in organisms ranging from yeast to mammals....dysregulation of insulin signaling and carbohydrate homeostasis in diabetes produces numerous aging-like symptoms including increased risk of cancer and other age-related diseases.

It's been over three years since that study was completed and no word has reached the media to tell the public about this finding. I ask myself why.

Even Glioblastoma is a product of glycation as explained in this report from Nov 2016 in PMC;

DISCUSSION

We investigated how the anti-neoplastic effect of carnosine is influenced by the nutritional supply of tumor cells and how glycolysis, the TCA cycle and OxPhos contribute to tumor cell survival. It was previously shown that pyruvate inhibits the anti-neoplastic effect of carnosine. We were thus interested to study, whether this can also be seen in glioblastoma tumor cells and whether the production of ATP via TCA cycle and OxPhos are responsible for this effect.

Keep in mind that glycolysis is what you get when you break down glucose. Think about what would happen if the glucose weren't there in the first place. Do you think the glioblastoma tumor could manifest?

Published Oct 12, 2016, the following report acknowledges that diet plays a large role in the formation of AGEs the single most important factor in cancer, as AGEs are at the root of all cancers;

- **The Role of Advanced_Glycation_End-Products in Cancer Disparity.**

Abstract

While the socioeconomic and environmental factors associated with cancer disparity have been well documented, the contribution of biological factors is an emerging field of research. Established disparity factors such as low income, poor diet, drinking alcohol, smoking, and a sedentary lifestyle may have molecular effects on the inherent biological makeup of the tumor itself, possibly altering cell signaling events and gene expression profiles to profoundly alter tumor development and progression. Our understanding of the molecular and biological consequences of poor lifestyle is lacking, but such information may significantly change how we approach goals to reduce cancer incidence and mortality rates within minority populations. In this review, we will summarize the biological, socioeconomic, and environmental associations between a group of reactive metabolites known as advanced glycation end-products (AGEs) and cancer health disparity. Due to their links with lifestyle and the activation of disease-associated pathways, AGEs may represent both a biological consequence and a bio-behavioral indicator of poor lifestyle which may be targeted within specific populations to reduce disparities in cancer incidence and mortality.

That means even brain cancer isn't immune to the effects of glycation. But that's not all, published at the end of last year was this report on the effects of HMGB1 on most all lung diseases;

- **Emerging role of HMGB1 in lung diseases: friend or foe.**

Abstract

Lung diseases remain a serious problem for public health. The immune status of the body is considered to be the main influencing factor for the progression of lung diseases. HMGB1 (high-mobility group box 1) emerges as an important molecule of the body immune network. Accumulating data have demonstrated that HMGB1 is crucially implicated in lung diseases and acts as an independent biomarker and therapeutic target for related lung diseases. This review provides an overview of updated understanding of HMGB1 structure, release styles, receptors, and function. Furthermore, we discuss the potential role of HMGB1 in a variety of lung diseases. Further exploration of molecular mechanisms underlying the function of HMGB1 in lung diseases will provide novel preventive and therapeutic strategies for lung diseases.

The following report details the overexpression of glycation in ovarian cancer. It was submitted Oct 28, 2016;

- **Overexpression of receptor for advanced glycation end products (RAGE) in ovarian cancer.**

Abstract

BACKGROUND:

Ovarian cancer is one of the important challenges in the field of gynecologic oncology because of some problems in understanding its etiology and pathogenesis. Receptor for advanced glycation end products (RAGE) is a multiligand trans-membranous receptor which is upregulated in some human cancers. Mechanisms of RAGE involvement in carcinogenesis of ovarian cancer are unknown.

OBJECTIVE:

This study aimed to investigate the expression of RAGE in ovarian cancers and its association with clinicopathological characteristics.

METHODS:

The RAGE expression level in ovarian cancer and corresponding noncancerous tissues were analyzed by real-time quantitative RT-PCR and immunohistochemistry techniques.

RESULTS:

Results indicated that RAGE gene was overexpressed in ovarian cancer tissue compared with adjacent noncancerous tissue ($p < 0.001$). A significant association between RAGE expression and tumor size ($p = 0.04$), depth of stromal invasion ($p = 0.031$), lymphovascular invasion ($p = 0.041$) and stage of cancer ($p = 0.041$) was observed. The receiver operating characteristic (ROC) analyses yielded the area under the curve (AUC) values of 0.86 for RAGE in discriminating ovarian cancer samples from non-cancer controls.

CONCLUSIONS:

In conclusion overexpression of RAGE in ovarian cancer may be a useful biomarker to predict tumor progression.

What interests me is that nothing is said about what creates these RAGEs. For thirty years they've been examining the nature of glycation but have said nothing about what is responsible for the major portion of glycation, glucose consumption in the form of sugar and grains. I guess that's not profitable.

What is profitable is finding more drugs to make people need more and more drugs. Evidenced here in this report dated Oct 23, 2014, yet nothing has been announced about this report, Did you hear about it?

- **RAGE is essential for oncogenic KRAS-mediated hypoxic signaling in pancreatic cancer.**

Abstract

A hypoxic tumor microenvironment is characteristic of many cancer types, including one of the most lethal, pancreatic cancer. We recently demonstrated that the receptor for advanced glycation end products (RAGE) has an important role in promoting the development of pancreatic cancer and attenuating the response to chemotherapy. We now demonstrate that binding of RAGE to oncogenic KRAS facilitates hypoxia-inducible factor 1 (HIF1)α activation and promotes pancreatic tumor growth under hypoxic conditions. Hypoxia induces NF-κB-dependent and HIF1α-independent RAGE expression in pancreatic tumor cells. Moreover, the interaction between RAGE and mutant KRAS increases under hypoxia, which in turn sustains KRAS signaling pathways (RAF-MEK-ERK and PI3K-AKT), facilitating stabilization and transcriptional activity of HIF1α. Knockdown of RAGE in vitro inhibits KRAS signaling, promotes HIF1α degradation, and increases hypoxia-induced pancreatic tumor cell death. RAGE-deficient mice have impaired oncogenic KRAS-driven pancreatic tumor growth with significant down-regulation of the HIF1α signaling pathway. Our results provide a novel mechanistic link between NF-κB, KRAS, and HIF1α, three potent molecular pathways in the cellular response to hypoxia during pancreatic tumor development and suggest alternatives for preventive and therapeutic strategies.

Obviously, the continuing need to examine the damage, instead of warning about the glycating substance proves to be more lucrative than realizing the actual cure, removing the glycating substances from the diet. Removing the glycating substances involves conquering an addiction, though. That wouldn't be too bad if this addiction wasn't inflicted on us. But it was, making this addiction almost impossible to conquer.

This study dated July 18, 2016, shows the influence of HMGB1 and M2 like macrophages in skin cancer;

- **Tumour hypoxia promotes melanoma growth and metastasis via High Mobility Group Box-1 and M2-like macrophages.**

Abstract

Hypoxia is a hallmark of cancer that is strongly associated with invasion, metastasis, resistance to therapy and poor clinical outcome. Tumour hypoxia affects immune responses and promotes the accumulation of macrophages in the tumor microenvironment. However, the signals linking tumor hypoxia to tumor-associated macrophage recruitment and tumor promotion are incompletely understood. Here we show that the damage-associated molecular pattern High-Mobility Group Box 1 protein (HMGB1) is released by melanoma tumor cells as a consequence of hypoxia and promotes M2-like tumor-associated macrophage accumulation and an IL-10 rich milieu within a tumor. Furthermore, we demonstrate that HMGB1 drives IL-10 production in M2-like macrophages by selectively signaling through the Receptor for Advanced Glycation End products (RAGE). Finally, we show that HMGB1 has an important role in murine B16 melanoma growth and metastasis, whereas in humans its serum concentration is significantly increased in metastatic melanoma. Collectively, our findings identify a mechanism by which hypoxia affects tumor growth and metastasis in melanoma and depict HMGB1 as a potential therapeutic target.

Stomach cancer is influenced as well by glycation as explained in this report submitted Oct 1, 2015;

- **Combined targeting of high-mobility group box-1 and interleukin-8 to control micro metastasis potential in gastric cancer.**

Abstract

Micrometastasis is the major cause of treatment failure in gastric cancer (GC). Because epithelial-to-mesenchymal transition (EMT) is considered to develop prior to macroscopic metastasis, EMT-promoting factors may affect micrometastasis. This study aimed to evaluate the role of extracellular high-mobility group box-1 (HMGB1) in EMT and the treatment effect of combined targeting of HMGB1 and interleukin-8 (IL-8) at early-stage GC progression through interrupting EMT promotion. Extracellular HMGB1 was induced by human recombinant HMGB1 and pCMV-SPORT6-HMGB1 plasmid transfection. EMT activation was evaluated by immunoblotting, immunofluorescence and immunohistochemistry. Increased migration/invasion activities were evaluated by in vitro transwell migration/invasion assay using all histological types of human GC cell lines (N87, MKN28 SNU-1, and KATOIII), N87-xenograft BALB/c nude mice and human paired serum-tissue GC samples. HMGB1-induced soluble factors were measured by chemiluminescent immunoassay. Inhibition effects of tumor growth and EMT activation by combined targeting of HMGB1 and IL-8 were evaluated in N87-xenograft nude mice. Serum HMGB1 increases along the GC carcinogenesis and reaches maximum before macroscopic metastasis. Overexpressed extracellular HMGB1 promoted EMT activation and increased cell motility/invasiveness through ligation to the receptor for advanced glycation end products. HMGB1-induced IL-8 overexpression contributed the HMGB1-induced EMT in GC in vitro and in vivo. Blocking HMGB1 caused significant reduction of tumor growth, and the addition of human recombinant IL-8 rescues this antitumor effects. Our results imply the role of HMGB1 in EMT through IL-8 mediation, and a potential mechanism of GC micrometastasis. Our observations suggest combination strategy of HMGB1 and IL-8 as a promising diagnostic and therapeutic target to control GC micrometastasis.

More evidence of Glycation in Breast cancer is in this report from Dec 23, 2016;

- **Accumulation of the advanced glycation end product carboxymethyl lysine in breast cancer is positively associated with estrogen receptor expression and unfavorable prognosis in estrogen receptor-negative cases.**

Abstract

Advanced glycation end products (AGEs) accumulate as a result of high concentrations of reactive aldehydes, oxidative stress, and insufficient degradation of glycated proteins. AGEs are therefore accepted biomarkers for aging, diabetes, and several degenerative diseases. Due to the Warburg effect and increased oxidative stress, cancer cells frequently accumulate significant amounts of AGEs. As the accumulation of AGEs may reflect the metabolic state and receptor signaling, we evaluated the potential prognostic and predictive value of this biomarker. We used immunohistochemistry to determine the AGE Nε-carboxymethyl-lysine (CML) in 213 mammary carcinoma samples and Western blotting to detect AGEs in cell cultures. Whereas no significant correlation between hormone receptor status and CML was observed in cell lines, CML accumulation in tumors was positively correlated with the presence of estrogen receptor alpha, the postmenopausal state, and age. A negative correlation was found for grade III carcinomas and triple-negative cases.

Again, this form of cancer can be curable if you remove the glycating factor. I have yet to find cancer that can't be cured by taking away the glycating factor, glucose. Why then is glucose still a recommended food, as in carbohydrates such as "whole grains"?

It amazes me how many studies they find to say the same thing over and over again. Yet they keep doing it, day after day after day, in an unending cycle of dependence. This report on the effects of RAGEs on esophageal and lung cancers;

- ***Tissue-specific expression profiling of receptor for advanced glycation end products and its soluble forms in esophageal and lung cancer.***

Abstract

The receptor for advanced glycation end products (RAGE) interacts with several ligands and is involved in various human diseases. Several splicing forms of the RAGE gene have been characterized, and two general mechanisms are usually responsible for the generation of soluble receptors. However, variants distribution and respective roles in different tumors are not clear. We analyzed RAGE and hRAGEsec mRNA expression in esophageal and lung cancer by RT-polymerase chain reaction. The Agilent clipper 1000 Bioanalyzer using lab-on-a-chip technology was applied to size and quantify the polymerase chain reaction products. Western blotting was performed to measure total soluble RAGE protein levels. The results showed that RAGE and its splice variants increased in esophageal cancers and decreased in lung cancers. We conclude that RAGE presents as a major isoform; soluble RAGE may also play certain roles in esophageal cancer and lung cancer.

How many reports does the FDA or the USDA need to tell them that what they're recommending for everyone to eat, is doing them more harm than good, far more?

This report dated June 15, 2007, shows the effects of AGEs on chondrosarcoma, a bone cancer;

- **Endogenous secretory receptor for advanced glycation endproducts as a novel prognostic marker in chondrosarcoma.**

Abstract

BACKGROUND:

Chondrosarcoma, the second most frequent primary malignant bone tumor, is classified into 3 grades according to histologic criteria of malignancy. However, a low-grade lesion can be difficult to distinguish from a benign enchondroma, whereas some histologically low-grade lesions may carry a poor prognosis. The receptor for advanced glycation endproducts (RAGE) and its ligand, high-mobility group box-1 (HMGB1), was quantified in enchondromas and chondrosarcomas to determine whether these markers were associated with histological malignancy and prognosis.

METHODS:

Enchondromas (n = 20) and typical chondrosarcomas (n = 39) were evaluated for RAGE, endogenous secretory RAGE (esRAGE, a splice variant form), and HMGB1 protein expression by immunohistochemistry including laser confocal microscopy. The content of esRAGE in resected specimens was measured with an enzyme-linked immunosorbent assay. Associations of these molecules with histology and clinical behavior of tumors were analyzed.

RESULTS:

Expression of esRAGE and HMGB1 was observed in all specimens. The numbers of cells positive for esRAGE and HMGB1 expression were positively associated with the histologic grade. Expression of esRAGE was significantly higher in chondrosarcomas than in enchondromas ($P < .001$). Tissue esRAGE content was also significantly higher in grade 1 and 2 chondrosarcomas than enchondromas ($P = .0255$ and $P = .008$, respectively). High expression of esRAGE in grade 1 chondrosarcoma was associated with subsequent recurrence ($P = .0013$), lung metastasis ($P = .0071$), and poor survival ($P < .001$).

CONCLUSIONS:

Assessment of esRAGE expression should aid in diagnostic and prognostic determinations in chondrosarcoma.

This report dated Nov 23, 2016, shows the effects that glycation and AGEs have on ovarian cancer and prostate cancer,

1. Introduction

Reactive oxygen species (ROS), generated as consequence of oxidative metabolism, activate signal transduction pathways, which contribute to cellular homeostasis. Metabolically active cells, neutrophils, and macrophages from the immune system produce high levels of ROS.

7. The Function of HMGB Proteins and Other Redox Sensors during Oxidative Stress in Ovarian Cancer

OS has been proposed as a cause of ovarian cancer. HMGB1 is considered a biomarker for ovarian cancer and increased levels of interleukin-8 protein (IL-8) and HMGB1 correlate with poor prognosis in prostate and ovarian cancer cells.

8. Oxidative Stress in Prostate Cancer and the Function of HMGB Proteins and Other Redox Sensors

The human prostate anatomy displays a zonal architecture, corresponding to central, periurethral transition, peripheral zone, and anterior fibromuscular stroma. The majority of prostate carcinomas are derived from the peripheral zone, while benign prostatic hyperplasia arises from the transition zone.

Finally, several research lines outline the direct importance of HMGB proteins in prostate cancer and their implications in therapy. Increased HMGB2 expression, HMGB1 expression, or coexpression of RAGE and HMGB1 has been associated with prostate cancer progression and has been correlated with poor patient outcome.

10. Conclusions and Perspectives

ROS overproduction and imbalance are a primary cause of malignancy in the onset of cancer. Cells have evolved multiple strategies in response to ROS production and HMGB proteins play a major role in many molecular mechanisms participating in these responses. In the nucleus, HMGB proteins affect DNA repair, transcription, and chromosomal stability; in the cytoplasm, they determine key decisions that finally lead towards autophagy or apoptosis; as extracellular signals, they produce changes that affect the microenvironment of a tumor and attract cells from the immune system. In turn, the inflammatory onset can increase ROS production and therefore enhances the response. HMGB1 and HMGB2 are expressed at the highest levels in immune cells and, besides, they have been related to cancers, which are hormone-responsive, such as ovarian and prostate cancers. Since HMGB proteins have many different functions and are necessary for healthy cells, an improved strategy to modulate their role in cancer progression could be to act through other proteins interacting specifically with them. The identification of HMGB partners, which could be univocally associated with specific cancerous processes or with the mechanism of cisplatin resistance, is a field of interest for ongoing translational cancer research. Interactive strategies are outstanding for the development of these research lines.

A search for cervical cancer and glycation returned 602 studies in the PMC index and started with this study;

- **Expression and Effects of High-Mobility Group Box 1 in Cervical Cancer**

We investigated the significance of high- mobility group box1 (HMGB1) and T-cell-mediated immunity and prognostic value in cervical cancer... The hmgb1 expression may activate Tregs or facilitate Th2 polarization to promote immune evasion of cervical cancer. Elevated HMGB1 protein in cervical carcinoma samples was associated with a high recurrence of HPV infection in univariate analysis... Data collected here demonstrated that the expression of HMGB1 in cervical lesions increased with tumor progression.

I wanted to see the relationship between glycation and bladder cancer. My search returned 616 studies, with the first one dated Feb 25, 2015;

- ***S100A12 and RAGE expression in human bladder transitional cell carcinoma: a role for the ligand/RAGE axis in tumor progression?***

CONCLUSIONS:

According to the results presented in the current study, mRNA expression of S100A12 and RAGE might be as a useful biomarker for TCC. Therefore, this ligand-receptor axis possibly plays important roles in the development of TCC and may serve either as an early diagnostic marker or as a key factor in the monitoring of response to treatment. More research is required concerning inhibition of the S100A12-RAGE axis in different cancer models.

Bladder cancer is the 4th most common cancer among men in the U.S. and more than half of patients experience recurrences within 5 years after initial diagnosis. Kidney disease isn't immune from the effects of glycation either, as expressed in this study from *Oct 29, 1993;*

- **Expression of receptors for** advanced glycosylation end products **on renal cell carcinoma cells in vitro.**

Abstract

Proteins that have been modified by long-term expose to glucose accumulate advanced glycosylation end products (AGEs) as a function of protein age. In these studies, we have examined the interaction of AGE-protein with renal cell carcinoma cells (RCC) in vitro, using AGE-modified bovine serum albumin (AGE-BSA) as a probe. AGE-BSA showed a tendency to induce in vitro cell growth of RCC cells and promoted the production of interleukin-6 (IL-6), an in vitro autocrine growth factor. Reverse transcriptase-polymerase chain reaction analysis revealed that RCC cells used here express mRNA for a receptor for AGEs (RAGE). These results suggested that AGEs taken up through RAGE on RCC cells might play a role in promoting the growth of RCC cells.

This was discovered in the summer of 1993 or prior, yet nothing was ever announced by the FDA or the USDA that there might be a preventative diet to protect against cancer. Did you hear anything about sugar or carbohydrates causing this kind of damage? I didn't. Yet the evidence is clear as day from a study done over 20 years ago. Still, nobody announced these revelations as they were being discovered. This report submitted Dec 2012;

- ***Functional amyloid formation by* STREPTOCOCCUS MUTANS**

In summary, there is a growing realization that amyloid formation is a directed, widespread, functional process that contributes to the biology of numerous micro-organisms, with particular relevance for adhesion and biofilm formation. We have now demonstrated amyloid formation by the cariogenic pathogen **S. MUTANS***, which is not surprising considering its biofilm niche. In addition to the contribution of amyloids to virulence by facilitating the adhesion, biofilm formation and invasion of pathogens, microbial amyloids have been postulated to contribute to systemic diseases, including Alzheimer's and Parkinson's, possibly by seeding amyloid formation in the brain.*

What's behind liver cancer? Copied from **PMC** on liver cancer;

According to the database from GLOBOCAN 2012, *liver cancer has the fifth highest incidence rate and is the second most life-threatening cancer in the world. There were an estimated 14.1 million new cases and 8.2 million cancer deaths worldwide in 2012, among which there were 782,500 new patients and 745,500 deaths caused by liver cancer.*

- **HMGB1 has been demonstrated as a critical role in a number of cancers, including colorectal, breast, lung, prostate, cervical, skin, kidney, gastric, pancreatic, osteosarcoma and leukemia.**

Recently, HMGB1 has been recognized as a pro-angiogenesis factor leading to the generation of vascular endothelial growth factor (VEGF) in colon cancer, while RAGE was identified as the requirement for cell angiogenesis in HCC (hepatocellular carcinoma).

Autophagy and apoptosis are recognized as both the programmed cell deaths. In HCC, the release of HMGB1 from nuclei to cytoplasm was reported as an inducer of autophagic cell death, which may be associated with ROS and/or Beclin-1.

*In summary, HMGB1 plays a pivotal role in oncogenesis and progression in HCC which may be a potential target for therapies and is worthy of further study. (*What's responsible for HMGB1?)

This free report appeared in PubMed 3/1/2016, it expresses the role AGEs and RAGE play in Colorectal cancer, yet it's been a year since this report and nothing's been publicized about this; (Again I ask myself why.)

- **Clinical significance of AGE-RAGE axis in colorectal cancer: associations with glyoxalase-I, adiponectin receptor expression, and prognosis.**

Abstract

BACKGROUND:

Advanced glycation end products (AGEs) and their receptor RAGE emerge as important pathogenic contributors in colorectal carcinogenesis. However, their relationship to the detoxification enzyme Glyoxalase (GLO)-I and Adiponectin receptors (AdipoR1, AdipoR2) in colorectal carcinoma (CRC) is currently understudied. In the present study, we investigated the expression levels of the above molecules in CRC compared to adjacent non-tumoral tissue and their potential correlation with clinicopathological characteristics and patients' survival.

METHODS:

We analyzed the immunohistochemical expression of AGE, RAGE and GLO-1, AdipoR1, and AdipoR2 in 133 primary CRC cases, focusing on GLO-1 The tumor MSI status was further assessed in mucinous carcinomas. Western immunoblotting was employed for validation of immunohistochemical data in normal and tumoral tissues as well as three CRC cell lines. An independent set of 55 patients was also used to validate the results of univariate survival analysis regarding GLO-1.

RESULTS:

CRC tissue showed the higher intensity of both AGE and RAGE expression compared with normal colonic mucosa which was negative for GLO-1 in most cases (78 %). Western immunoblotting confirmed AGE, RAGE and GLO-1 overexpression in tumoral tissue. GLO-1 expression was directly related to RAGE and inversely related to AGE immunolabeling. There was a trend towards higher expression of all markers (except for RAGE) in the subgroup of mucinous carcinomas which, although of borderline significance, seemed to be more prominent for AdipoR1 and AGE. Additionally, AGE, AdipoR1, and Adipo R2 expression were related to tumor grade, whereas GLO-1 and AdipoR1 to T-category. In survival analysis, AdipoR2 and GLO-1 overexpression predicted shortened survival in the entire cohort and in early-stage cases, an effect which for GLO-1 was reproduced in the validation cohort. Moreover, GLO-1 emerged as an independent prognosticator of adverse significance in the patients' cohort.

CONCLUSIONS:

We herein provide novel evidence regarding the possible interactions between the components of the AGE-RAGE axis, GLO-1 and adiponectin receptors in CRC. AGE and AdipoR1 are possibly involved in colorectal carcinogenesis, whereas AdipoR2 and GLO-1 emerged as novel independent prognostic biomarkers of adverse significance for patients with early disease stage. Further studies are warranted to extend our observations and investigate their potential therapeutic significance.

I'll bet that you thought that esophageal cancer was the result of smoking only. My best friend lost his wife to esophageal cancer 30 years ago. This study shows that it's not just the smoke that causes this cancer. Glycation of carbs tends to promote this cancer just as much as the smoking.

- **Plasma miR-185 is decreased in patients with esophageal squamous cell carcinoma and might suppress tumor migration and invasion by targeting RAGE.**

The receptor for advanced-glycation end products (RAGE) is upregulated in various cancers and has been associated with tumor progression, but little is known about its expression and regulation by microRNAs (miRNAs) in esophageal squamous cell carcinoma (ESCC). Here, we describe miR-185, which represses RAGE expression and investigate the biological role of miR-185 in ESCC. In this study, we found that the high level of RAGE expression in 29 pairs of paraffin-embedded ESCC tissues was correlated positively with the depth of invasion by immunohistochemistry, suggesting that RAGE was involved in ESCC. We used bioinformatics searches and luciferase reporter assays to investigate the prediction that RAGE was regulated directly by miR-185. Besides, overexpression of miR-185 in ESCC cells was accompanied by 27% (TE-11) and 49% (Eca-109) reduced RAGE expression. The effect was further confirmed in RAGE protein by immunofluorescence in both cell lines. The effects were reversed following cotransfection with miR-185 and high-level expression of the RAGE vector. Furthermore, the biological role of miR-185 in ESCC cell lines was investigated using assays of cell viability, Ki-67 staining, and cell migration and invasion, as well as in a xenograft model. We found that overexpression of miR-185 inhibited migration and invasion by ESCC cells in vitro and reduced their capacity to develop distal pulmonary metastases in vivo partly through the RAGE/heat shock protein 27 pathway. Interestingly, in clinical specimens, the level of plasma miR-185 expression was decreased significantly ($P = 0.002$) in patients with ESCC [0.500; 95% confidence interval (CI) 0.248-1.676] compared with healthy controls (2.410; 95% CI 0.612-5.671). The value of the area under the receiver-operating characteristic curve was 0.73 (95% CI 0.604-0.855). In conclusion, our findings shed novel light on the role of miR-185/RAGE in ESCC metastasis, and plasma miR-185 has potential as a novel diagnostic biomarker in ESCC.

Are these enough reports to prove how glycation directly influence cancer? After reading this can you see the logic in controlling cancer by controlling your carb intake? Where are the warnings from the FDA and the USDA? Don't they care about what they're recommending? Don't they understand, because of their recommendations, they send millions of Moms and Dads, sisters and brothers, husbands and wives to their slow, expensive, painful deaths?

These are free reports that are available to everyone. All you have to do is search for them at the National Library of Medicine in the National Institute of Health. There are literally 100s of thousands of reports on the effects of glycation that remain hidden in the PubMed and PMC databases except to the few who look through them. The only ones looking through this database are the drug companies looking for more ways to make money. Nobody is looking to warn anyone of the dangers of this food.

My question is why? The answer I get is, "there's no money in it". That's is why I said in my first book, it would be a shame if profits and money weren't the primary motivating factors in our society, but they are, and we have to live with it. That's why I choose not to buy into it. You have the same choice.

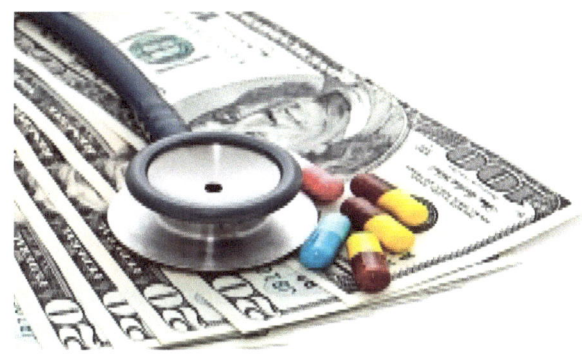

HEART TO HEART HERE'S YOUR KEY

TO LIFELONG HEALTH FOR ETERNITY

CURB YOUR CARBS WHILE YOU STILL CAN

AND END THAT PAIN THAT CARBS DEMAND

Chapter 6
Can Your Type of Heart Disease be Cured or Just Treated?

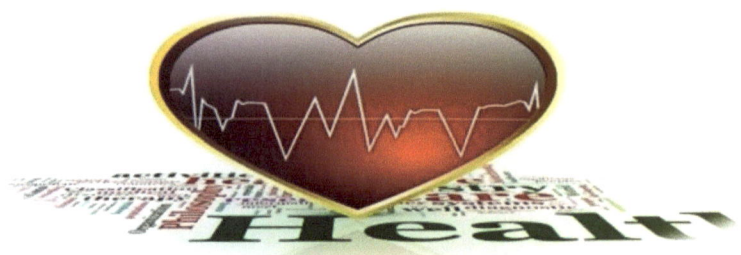

This chapter has been reserved for atherosclerosis and other heart-related diseases. Dementias and diseases of inflammation will be in the next chapter, as well with all other disorders that inflammation is responsible for.

Listed below from PubMed or PMC or the FDA are reports of studies done on the effects of glycation and its influence in any CVD or disease influenced by inflammation, which is a direct cause of glycation.

- ***Advanced glycation endproducts induce apoptosis of endothelial progenitor cells by activating receptor RAGE and NADPH oxidase/JNK signaling axis.***

Elevated levels of advanced glycation endproducts (AGEs) is an important risk factor for atherosclerosis. Dysfunction of endothelial progenitor cells (EPCs), which is essential for re-endothelialization and neovascularization, is a hallmark of atherosclerosis. However, it remains unclear whether and how AGEs acts on EPCs to promote the pathogenesis of atherosclerosis. In this study, EPCs were exposed to different concentrations of AGEs. The expression of NADPH and Rac1 was measured to investigate the involvement of NADPH oxidase pathway. ROS was examined to indicate the level of oxidative stress in EPCs. Total JNK and p-JNK were determined by Western blotting. Cell apoptosis was evaluated by both TUNEL staining and flow cytometry. Cell proliferation was measured by (3)H thymidine uptake. The results showed that treatment of EPCs with AGEs increased the levels of ROS in EPCs. Mechanistically, AGEs increased the activity of NADPH oxidase and the expression of Rac1, a major component of NADPH. Importantly, treatment of EPCs with AGEs activated the JNK signaling pathway, which was closely associated with cell apoptosis and inhibition of proliferation. Our results suggest that the RAGE activation by AGEs in EPCs upregulates intracellular ROS levels, which contributes to the increased activity of NADPH oxidase and expression of Rac1, thus promoting cellular apoptosis and inhibiting proliferation. Mechanistically, AGEs binding to the receptor RAGE in EPCs is associated with hyperactivity of JNK signaling pathway, which is downstream of ROS. Our findings suggest that dysregulation of the AGEs/RAGE axis in EPCs may promote atherosclerosis and identify the NADPH/ROS/JNK signaling axis as a potential target for therapeutic intervention.

With the list growing past 17,729 studies on the effects of glycation, I think this message about the process of glycation should be wider known. This is the basis of all modern disease. Why has it been kept hidden? Is it due to industrial concerns? What would happen to the pharmaceutical/chemical industry if you wiped 98% of all illness?

This report dictates how the modification of proteins (glycation) is involved in atherosclerosis. This is the smoking gun that carbs are dangerous foods to eat. Even though this report is from Dec 2016, it only says, again, what hundreds if not thousands of other reports dictate. They all dictate glycation is dangerous. What causes glycation should be avoided at all costs, to ensure optimal health.

- **Cellular mechanisms and consequences of glycation in atherosclerosis and obesity.**

Post-translational modification of proteins imparts diversity to protein functions. The process of glycation represents a complex set of pathways that mediate advanced glycation endproduct (AGE) formation, detoxification, intracellular disposition, extracellular release, and induction of signal transduction. These processes modulate the response to hyperglycemia, obesity, aging, inflammation, and renal failure, in which AGE formation and accumulation are facilitated. It has been shown that endogenous anti-AGE protective mechanisms are thwarted in chronic disease, thereby amplifying accumulation and detrimental cellular actions of these species. Atop these considerations, receptor for advanced glycation endproducts (RAGE)-mediated pathways downregulate expression and activity of the key anti-AGE detoxification enzyme, glyoxalase-1 (GLO1), thereby setting in motion an interminable feed-forward loop in which AGE-mediated cellular perturbation is not readily extinguished. In this review, we consider recent work in the field highlighting roles for glycation in obesity and atherosclerosis and discuss emerging strategies to block the adverse consequences of AGEs. This article is part of a Special Issue entitled: The role of post-translational protein modifications on the heart and vascular metabolism edited by Jason R.B. Dyck & Jan F.C. Glatz.

If this is the smoking gun that proves what glucose consumption does to the body in the form of atherosclerosis, how long before the FDA or the USDA will admit that this is what happens after ingesting grains? Will the Heart Association say anything about this? What about the American Diabetic Association? I wonder if this news will reach any regulatory agency. My guess is because Monsanto has something to say about it, any regulatory agency will say what Monsanto wants them to say, as they're mostly all controlled by Monsanto.

This report from Aug 1, 1989, reveals how aware we were then, that glycation as a damaging process, is caused by excess glucose in your system. One would think that 28 years would be long enough to reveal this information. Apparently, it wasn't. But now you know:

- *Nonenzymatic glycation of human blood platelet proteins.*

We studied 11 diabetic patients, all of whom had the severe atherothrombotic disease, and 11 normal controls. Overall glycation was assessed by the extent of incorporation of [3H]-NaBH4 into fructose lysine separated from whole platelet proteins following amino acid analysis. Fructosyl lysine represented 5.7% +/- 1.0 S.D. of the total radioactivity in the normal whole platelet samples. Increased glycation was observed in platelets from 5 of the 11 diabetics. Platelet glycation did not correlate with glycation of hemoglobin or albumin. The pattern of glycation of various platelet proteins in whole platelets, as determined by the incorporation of [3H]-NaBH4 into electrophoretically separated proteins did not display selectivity, although myosin and glycoproteins IIb and IIIa showed relatively increased levels of [3H]-NaBH4 incorporation. Artificially glycated platelet membranes exhibited glycation mainly in proteins corresponding to the electrophoretic mobility of myosin, glycoproteins IIb, and IIIa.

The previous report was published in 1989, yet have you heard anything about it? Didn't they any have an idea, at that time, what carbs were doing to the body, when ingested? I guess they needed more studies. Over 17,000 of them have been filed as of yet. Why has it taken until 2010 to learn any of this? Even today, they still are reluctant to admit such, that carbs are dangerous foods to be eating.

- **Advanced glycation end products: An emerging biomarker for adverse outcome in patients with peripheral artery disease.**

Patients with peripheral artery disease (PAD) suffer from widespread atherosclerosis. Partly due to the growing awareness of cardiovascular disease, the incidence of PAD has increased considerably during the past decade. It is anticipated that algorithms to identify high-risk patients for cardiovascular events require being updated, making use of novel biomarkers. Advanced glycation end products (AGEs) are moieties (elements) formed non-enzymatically on long-lived proteins under influence of glycemic and oxidative stress reactions. We elaborate on the formation and effects of AGEs, and the methods to measure AGEs. Several studies have been performed with AGEs in PAD. In this review, we evaluate the emerging evidence of AGEs as a clinical biomarker for patients with PAD.

Peripheral Artery disease is often the start of Atherosclerosis and all CVDs. They are a direct cause of glycation. Glycation is controllable by controlling the number of carbs you put in your mouth every time you eat.

This following study shows how your body reacts to the glucose infusion by sending out macrophages to counteract the damage presented by the glucose. The modified LDL particles are the glycated endproducts of what happens to your cholesterol with glucose in your system.

- **How do macrophages sense modify low-density lipoproteins?**

Abstract

In atherosclerosis, serum lipoproteins undergo various chemical modifications that impair their normal function. Modification of low-density lipoprotein (LDL) such as oxidation, glycation, carbamylation, glucooxidation, etc. makes LDL particles more proatherogenic. Macrophages are responsible for clearance of modified LDL to prevent cytotoxicity, tissue injury, inflammation, and metabolic disturbances. They develop an advanced sensing arsenal composed of various pattern recognition receptors (PRRs) capable of recognizing and binding foreign or altered-self targets for further inactivation and degradation. Modified LDL can be sensed and taken up by macrophages with a battery of scavenger receptors (SRs), of which SR-A1, CD36, and LOX1 play a major role. However, in atherosclerosis, lipid balance is deregulated that induces inability of macrophages to completely recycle modified LDL and leads to lipid deposition and transformation of macrophages to foam cells. SRs also mediate various pathogenic effects of modified LDL on macrophages through activation of the intracellular signaling network. Other PRRs such Toll-like receptors can also interact with modified LDL and mediate their effects independently or in cooperation with SRs.

What you should think about, is what would happen if the glucose weren't there? The cholesterol can do what it's supposed to do, feed your body.

From Dec 2016, Coronary Heart Disease and Ischemic stroke are shown to be influenced by another RAGE Gly82ser. How many more of these do they have to find before they realize that you can prevent this by keeping carbs out of the diet?

- **Association of RAGE gene Gly82Ser polymorphism with coronary artery disease and ischemic stroke: A systematic review and meta-analysis.**

Abstract

BACKGROUND:

The receptor for advanced glycosylation end products (RAGE) has been widely linked to diabetic atherosclerosis, but its effects on coronary artery disease (CAD) and ischemic stroke (IS) remain controversial. The Gly82Ser polymorphism is located in the ligand-binding V domain of RAGE, suggesting a possible influence of this variant on RAGE function. The aim of the present study is to clarify the association between the RAGE Gly82Ser polymorphism and susceptibility to CAD and IS.

CONCLUSIONS:

The current meta-analysis suggests that the RAGE Gly82Ser polymorphism is associated with an increased risk of CAD and IS, especially in the Chinese population. However, better-designed studies with larger sample sizes are needed to validate the results.

The following report submitted Sep 31, 2011, shows the influence of RAGE in VRD;

- **RAGE-dependent activation of the oncoprotein Pim1 plays a critical role in systemic vascular remodeling processes.**

Abstract

OBJECTIVE:

Vascular remodeling diseases (VRD) are mainly characterized by inflammation and vascular smooth muscle cells (VSMCs) proliferative an anti-apoptotic phenotype. Recently, the activation of the advanced glycation endproducts receptor (RAGE) has been shown to promote VSMC proliferation and resistance to apoptosis in VRD in a signal transducer and activator of transcription (STAT)3-dependent manner. Interestingly, we previously described in both cancer and VRD that the sustainability of this proliferative and antiapoptotic phenotype requires activation of the transcription factor NFAT (nuclear factor of activated T-cells). In cancer, NFAT activation is dependent on the oncoprotein provirus integration site for Moloney murine leukemia virus (Pim1), which is regulated by STAT3 and activated in VRD. Therefore, we hypothesized that RAGE/STAT3 activation in VSMC activates Pim1, promoting NFAT and thus VSMC proliferation and resistance to apoptosis. Methods/Results- In vitro, freshly isolated human carotid VSMCs exposed to RAGE activator Nε-(carboxymethyl)lysine (CML) for 48 hours had (1) activated STAT3 (increased P-STAT3/STAT3 ratio and P-STAT3 nuclear translocation); (2) increased STAT3-dependent Pim1 expression resulting in NFATc1 activation; and (3) increased Pim1/NFAT-dependent VSMC proliferation (PCNA, Ki67) and resistance to mitochondrial-dependent apoptosis (TMRM, Annexin V, TUNEL). Similarly to RAGE inhibition (small interfering RNA [siRNA]), Pim1, STAT3 and NFATc1 inhibition (siRNA) reversed these abnormalities in human carotid VSMC. Moreover, carotid artery VSMCs isolated from Pim1 knockout mice were resistant to CML-induced VSMC proliferation and resistance to apoptosis. In vivo, RAGE inhibition decreases STAT3/Pim1/NFAT activation, reversing vascular remodeling in the rat carotid artery-injured model.

CONCLUSIONS:

RAGE activation accounts for many features of VRD including VSMC proliferation and resistance to apoptosis by the activation of the STAT3/Pim1/NFAT axis. Molecules aimed to inhibit RAGE could be of a great therapeutic interest for the treatment of VRD.

Advanced glycation end products increase lipids accumulation in macrophages through upregulation of receptor of advanced glycation end products: increasing uptake, esterification and decreasing efflux of cholesterol.

BACKGROUND:

Previous reports have suggested that advanced glycation end products (AGEs) participate in the pathogenesis of diabetic macroangiopathy. Our *previous study has found that AGEs can increase the lipid droplets accumulation in aortas of diabetic rats, but the current understanding of the mechanisms remains incomplete by which AGEs affect lipids accumulation in macrophages and accelerate atherosclerosis. In this study, we investigated the role of AGEs on lipids accumulation in macrophages and the possible molecular mechanisms including cholesterol influx, esterification, and efflux of macrophages.*

METHODS:

THP-1 cells were incubated with PMA to differentiate to be macrophages which were treated with AGEs in the concentration of 300 µg/ml and 600 µg/ml with or without anti-RAGE (receptor for AGEs) antibody and then stimulated by oxidized-LDL (ox-LDL) or Dil-ox-LDL. Lipids accumulation was examined by oil red staining. The cholesterol uptake, esterification, and efflux were detected respectively by fluorescence microscope, enzymatic assay kit, and fluorescence microplate. Quantitative RT-PCR and Western blot were used to measure the expression of the molecular involved in cholesterol uptake, synthesis/esterification, and efflux.

RESULTS:

AGEs increased lipids accumulation in macrophages in a concentration-dependent manner. 600 µg/ml AGEs obviously upregulated oxLDL uptake, increased levels of cholesterol ester in macrophages, and decreased the HDL-mediated cholesterol efflux by regulating the main molecular expression including CD36, Scavenger receptors (SR) A2, HMG-CoA reductase (HMGCR), ACAT1 and ATP-binding cassette transporter G1 (ABCG1). The changes above were inverted when the cells were pretreated with the anti-RAGE antibody.

CONCLUSIONS:

The current study suggests that AGEs can increase lipids accumulation in macrophages by regulating cholesterol uptake, esterification and efflux mainly through binding with RAGE, which provide a deep understanding of mechanisms how AGEs accelerating diabetic atherogenesis.

This is the proof that AGEs inhibit proper cell nutrition by preventing the flow of cholesterol into the cell. This allows accumulation of LDL particles in your blood. Usually, with a carbohydrate diet, those LDL particles are going to be ApoB particles and those are the most proliferate in all disease. Again, this is something you have full control over, as you don't have to eat this food. There are plenty of healthier alternatives.

The next study details how *glycol-AGEs* work their way into the cellular wall of your arteries creating Atherosclerosis. What you should think about, does this always happen with glucose in your system? Can you live without glucose? If you answered YES to both of those questions, you're on your way understanding how to make your body healthier.

- **Glycolaldehyde-derived advanced glycation end products (glycol-AGEs)-induced vascular smooth muscle cell** *dysfunction is regulated by the AGES-receptor (RAGE) axis in endothelium.*

Advanced glycation end-products (AGEs) are involved in the development of vascular smooth muscle cell (VSMC) dysfunction and the progression of atherosclerosis. However, AGEs may indirectly affect VSMCs via AGEs-induced signal transduction between monocytes and human umbilical endothelial cells (HUVECs), rather than having a direct influence. This study was designed to elucidate the signaling pathway underlying AGEs-RAGE axis influence on VSMC dysfunction using a co-culture system with monocytes, HUVECs and VSMCs. AGEs stimulated the production of reactive oxygen species and pro-inflammatory mediators such as tumor necrosis factor-α and interleukin-1β via extracellular-signal-regulated kinases phosphorylation and nuclear factor-κB activation in HUVECs. It was observed that AGEs-induced pro-inflammatory cytokines increase VSMC proliferation, inflammation and vascular remodeling in the co-culture system. This result implies that RAGE plays a role in AGEs-induced VSMC dysfunction. We suggest that the regulation of signal transduction via the AGEs-RAGE axis in the endothelium can be a therapeutic target for preventing atherosclerosis.

Do you have any idea of how to regulate the transduction of AGEs? It's simple, go keto. Will an industry that depends on your illness, tell you that? I seriously doubt it. Since it's this industry that regulates the regulatory agencies, I doubt that you'll ever hear it from them. That's why it's so important to follow your own advice to stay healthy, stay away from unhealthy substances. Now you know how unhealthy glucose is, simply due to its glycative effects.

If you need more reports to prove how glucose directly influence heart disease, there are literally thousands of them. After reading them, it's easier see the logic in controlling your cardiovascular disease by controlling your carb intake? Where are the warnings from the FDA and the USDA? Don't they care about what they're recommending? Don't they understand because of their recommendations, they send millions of Moms and Dads, sisters, and brothers, husbands and wives to their slow, expensive, painful deaths?

These are free reports that are available to everyone. All you have to do is search for them at the National Library of Medicine in the National Institute of Health. There are literally 100s of thousands of reports on the effects of glycation that remain hidden in the PubMed and PMC databases except to the few who look through them. The only ones looking through this database are the drug companies looking for more ways to make money. Nobody is looking to warn anyone of the dangers of this food.

My question is why? The answer I get is, "there's no money in it". That's is why I said in my first book, it would be a shame if profits and money weren't the primary motivating factors in our society, but they are, and we have to live with it. That's why I choose not to buy into it. It's the same choice you have.

Chapter 7

Can Your Dementia, Osteoporosis, IBS/IBD, Asthma or Other Disease of Inflammation be Cured or Just Treated?

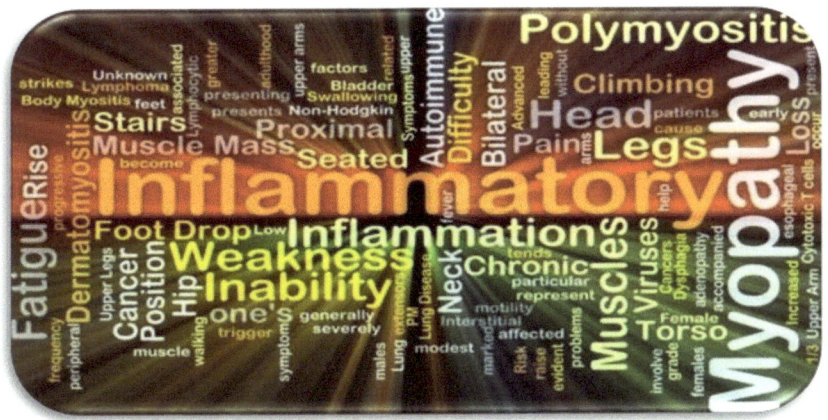

This poses an interesting question, osteoporosis, and dementia have something in common? Yes, they do. They are diseases of inflammation and inflammation is a product of glycation. It's these glycative cytokines and plaques that are responsible for all the damage that creates all diseases of inflammation. They are also responsible for IBS/IBD, Lupus, Fibromyalgia, Psoriasis, COPD, and every other disease that is influenced by inflammation, which would include most heart diseases and cancer.

Unfortunately, like arthritis, much of the damage has already been done and can't be undone. However, you can stop the decline immediately and start some recovery. Just realize that the recovery will take twice as long as it took for you to create this quagmire of disease in the first place. That only means that you must stop the glycation as soon as possible. (I suggest immediately, with a 3-day water only fast.) This will give your body more time to repair the damage.

Since the body needs proteins and cholesterol to operate and doesn't need the sugar, that leaves only one type of food to be responsible for glycation, carbs. I've learned through my research that the body can create all the glucose it needs with a process called gluconeogenesis. Gluconeogenesis is a process your body goes through whenever is needs glucose and has none readily available.

It produces this glucose with your own glycogen. That's what your body turns glucose into when you eat sugar and carbs. That is what makes me question our need to eat glucose. If your body can create what it needs, why eat it? You can live perfectly well without it because your body can make it.

Why then, where we fed the line, for 50 years that we had to make grains (the foundation of glucose in the body) the largest part of our diet? Could it be because these studies started about 60 years ago? They intensified 30 years ago when Monsanto took over GD Searle pharmaceuticals. This was also about the time when the whole grain ruse started convincing the public to consume massive amounts of this carcinogenic, atherosclerotic, inflammatory food. Do you wonder now, why all the disease exists?

When you cure a disease, you have nothing to treat. Where's the money flow in our medical industry? It flows through the treatment process. Every hospital proves this, every weight loss clinic proves this, every orthopedic clinic proves this. Actually, every clinic proves this. If a cure was found for all modern disease, what would it do to the health and medical industries? Reduce it to treating emergencies only? In another chapter of this book, I show you how reducing carb consumption will reduce emergencies as well. (That's where this really gets good.) It has something to do with its effect on your emotions.

Listed below from PubMed or PMC or the FDA are reports of studies done on the effects of glycation and its influence in osteoporosis or any disease influenced by inflammation.

Enzymes affecting your emotions are influenced by these foods affecting inflammation as well as cancer, which I've listed here. Probably the first condition to hit you will be IBS or IBD, Irritable Bowel Syndrome or Inflammatory Bowel Disease. This was just submitted this year in Feb;

- ***Prevalence and Impact of Inflammatory Bowel Disease-Irritable Bowel Syndrome on Patient-reported Outcomes in CCFA Partners.***

Abstract

BACKGROUND:

Inflammatory bowel disease (IBD) patients with persistent symptoms despite no or minimal inflammation are frequently described as having an overlap of IBD and irritable bowel syndrome (IBD-IBS). Limited data are available on how IBS impacts the individual patient with IBD. In this study, we aimed to evaluate the prevalence of IBD-IBS and investigate its impact on patient-reported outcomes.

METHOD:

We performed a cross-sectional analysis of the CCFA Partners Study. Bivariate analyses and logistic regression models were used to investigate associations between IBD-IBS and various demographic, disease factors, and patient-reported outcomes including anxiety, depression, sleep disturbances, pain interference, and social satisfaction.

RESULTS:

Of the 6309 participants included, a total of 1279 (20%) reported a coexisting IBS diagnosis. The prevalence of IBD-IBS in this cohort was similar within disease subtypes. A diagnosis of IBD-IBS was associated with higher narcotic use compared with those with no IBS diagnosis for both Crohn's disease, 17% versus 11% ($P < 0.001$) and ulcerative colitis/indeterminate colitis, 9% versus 5% ($P < 0.001$). Quality of life, as measured by Short Inflammatory Bowel Disease Questionnaire (SIBDQ) was lower in patients with IBD-IBS compared with those without. IBD-IBS diagnosis was associated with anxiety, depression, fatigue, sleep disturbances, pain interference, and decreased social satisfaction.

CONCLUSIONS:

In this sample of patients with IBD, the high prevalence of concomitant IBS diagnosis was observed. IBD-IBS diagnosis was associated with increased narcotic use and adverse patient-reported outcome. Appropriate diagnosis, treatment, and counseling may help improve the functional status of IBD-IBS patients and decrease narcotic use.

My appropriate treatment for this disorder isn't a treatment. Those always lead to more treatments. I propose a cure. All the inflammation involved in these disorders can be controlled by your intake of carbs, meaning, by going keto you can avoid all inflammation. How far do you think would that go to providing you relief from your pain?

- **Novel Insights into the Relationship between Diabetes and Osteoporosis**

Abstract

Only three decades ago adipose tissue was considered inert with little relationship to insulin resistance. Similarly, bone has long been thought purely in its structural context. In the last decade, emerging evidence has revealed important endocrine roles for both bone and adipose tissue. The interaction between these two tissues is remarkable. Bone marrow mesenchymal stem cells give rise to both osteoblasts and adipocytes. Leptin and adiponectin, two adipokines secreted by fat tissue, control energy homeostasis, but also have complex actions on the skeleton. In turn, the activities of bone cells are not limited to their bone remodeling activities, but also to modulation of adipose sensitivity and insulin secretion. This review will discuss these new insights linking bone remodeling to the control of fat metabolism and the association between diabetes mellitus and osteoporosis.

Conclusion

Chronic hyperglycemia profoundly affects multiple tissues and directly affects the frequency of complications in diabetes mellitus. Hypoinsulinemia is the primary hormonal disturbance leading to T1DM, whereas insulin resistance causing hyperglycemia is the principal event in T2DM. As discussed, bone mineral density is a relatively poor surrogate for defining bone structure during long-standing hyperglycemia. Low bone mass is often detected in T1DM although the pathogenesis is likely to be multifactorial. On the other hand, BMD can be low, normal or increased in T2DM. Yet both forms of diabetes are associated with an increased risk of fracture. In part, higher rates of fracture can be related to neuropathic, nephropathic and retinopathic changes that lead to a greater risk of falling. In addition, low body weight, hypoinsulinemia, low serum levels of IGF-I and altered gonadal steroids favor a catabolic state in the skeleton of Type I diabetics. The presence of obesity and T2DM, although associated with increased cortical bone mass, does not translate to a lower fracture risk, and paradoxically may enhance risk. Hyperglycemia can lead to degenerative changes in bone quality through advanced end product glycation, which particularly affects collagen cross-linking. Not surprisingly, one of the classic late clinical features of diabetes mellitus, i.e. vascular calcification, is associated with lower bone mass and impaired bone strength. Those two processes may be linked to reduced renal function and aberrant deposition of calcium in blood vessels rather than in the appropriate collagen matrix. Notwithstanding the potential numerous insults associated with sustained hyperglycemia, several recent developments suggest there is now a greater awareness of the skeleton as both a target of diabetic complications and a potential pathogenetic factor in the disease itself.*

Could this indicate that it might be healthier to feed your kids fats and proteins instead of carbs, to help save them from broken bones? How about yourself?

The following study looked at the brains of Alzheimer's disease patients. It's dated Jan 3, 2017. They officially label Alzheimer's disease as type 3 diabetes;

- *Type 3 Diabetes Mellitus: A Novel Implication of Alzheimer Disease.*

Abstract

The brain of patients with Alzheimer disease (AD) showed the evidence of reduced expression of insulin and neuronal insulin receptors, as compared with those of age-matched controls. This event gradually and certainly leads to a breakdown of the entire insulin-signaling pathway, which manifests insulin resistance. This, in turn, affects brain metabolism and cognitive functions, which are the best-documented abnormalities in the AD. These observations led Dr. de la Monte and her colleagues to suggest that AD is actually a neuroendocrine disorder that resembles type 2 diabetes mellitus. The truth would be more complex with understanding the role of Aβ derived diffusible ligands, advanced glycation end products, and low-density lipoprotein receptor-related protein 1. However, now it's known as "brain diabetes" and is called type 3 diabetes mellitus (T3DM). This review provides an overview of "brain diabetes" focusing on the reason why the phenomenon is called T3DM.

Evidence of inflammation's role in myasthenia gravis, dated Jan 3, 2017; I used to have a granddaughter with myasthenia gravis, as I recall at that time, there was no known cause. I guess the cause wasn't known then. It's a nice thing to know that it is now, but who are suggesting that we remove the instigating factor from this equation, the glucose that is responsible for the glycation? It's nicer to realize that there are a growing number of us;

- **Profile of upregulated inflammatory proteins in sera of Myasthenia Gravis patients.**

Abstract

This study describes specific patterns of elevated inflammatory proteins in clinical subtypes of myasthenia gravis (MG) patients. MG is a chronic, autoimmune neuromuscular disease with antibodies most commonly targeting the acetylcholine receptors (AChRab), which causes fluctuating skeletal muscle fatigue. MG pathophysiology includes a strong component of inflammation and a large proportion of patients with early onset MG additionally present thymus hyperplasia. Due to the fluctuating nature and heterogeneity of the disease, there is a great need for objective biomarkers as well as novel potential inflammatory targets. We examined the sera of 45 MG patients (40 AChRab seropositive and 5 AChRab seronegative), investigating 92 proteins associated with inflammation. Eleven of the analysed proteins were significantly elevated compared to healthy controls, out of which the three most significant were: matrix metalloproteinase 10 (MMP-10; $p = 0.0004$), transforming growth factor alpha (TGF-α; $p = 0.0017$) and extracellular newly identified receptor for advanced glycation end-products binding protein (EN-RAGE) (also known as protein S100-A12; $p = 0.0054$). Further, levels of MMP-10, C-X-C motif ligand 1 (CXCL1) and brain-derived neurotrophic factor (BDNF) differed between early and late onset MG. These novel targets provide valuable additional insight into the systemic inflammatory response in MG.

Do you worry about kidney disease? This report from May 2017 shows what's behind it;

- **Inflammation, oxidative stress, apoptosis, and autophagy in diabetes mellitus and diabetic kidney disease: the Four Horsemen of the Apocalypse.**

- *Abstract*

Diabetic kidney disease (DKD) can occur in approximately 30-40% of both type 1 and type 2 diabetic patients. The well-established features of DKD include increased serum glucose levels along with chronic low-grade inflammation, OxS, increased advanced glycation end products, sorbitol accumulation, increased hexosamine, and protein kinase C pathway activation. On the other hand, accumulating evidence suggests that novel pathways including apoptosis and autophagy might also play important roles in the pathogenesis and progression of DKD. In this review, the integrated mechanisms of inflammation, oxidative stress, apoptosis, and autophagy are discussed in the pathogenesis as well as the progression of DM and DKD.

This following report dated Feb 2017 shows the importance of sRAGE involved in lung infections and other inflammatory precursors to lung cancer;

- **The shedding-derived soluble receptor for advanced glycation endproducts sustains inflammation during acute Pseudomonas aeruginosa lung infection.**

Abstract

BACKGROUND:

The membrane-bound isoform of the receptor for advanced glycation end products (FL-RAGE) is primarily expressed by alveolar epithelial cells and undergoes shedding by the protease ADAM10, giving rise to soluble cleaved RAGE (cRAGE). RAGE has been associated with the pathogenesis of several acute and chronic lung disorders. Whether the proteolysis of FL-RAGE is altered by a given inflammatory stimulus is unknown. Pseudomonas aeruginosa causes nosocomial infections in hospitalized patients and is the major pathogen associated with chronic lung diseases.

CONCLUSIONS:

These data are the first to suggest that inhibition of FL-RAGE shedding, by affecting the FL-RAGE/cRAGE levels, is a novel mechanism for controlling inflammation to acute P. aeruginosa pneumonia. sRAGE in the alveolar space sustains inflammation in this setting.

Wonder where your backache came from? Did you think it was from standing all day or lifting something heavy? Think again, here's your proof that IVDD, intervertebral disk disease is created by nothing but than glycation. This report from Nov 2016;

- **AGEs induce ectopic endochondral ossification in intervertebral discs**

Abstract

Ectopic calcifications in intervertebral discs (IVDs) are known characteristics of IVD degeneration that are not commonly reported but may be implicated in structural failure and dysfunctional IVD cell metabolic responses. This study investigated the novel hypothesis that ectopic calcifications in the IVD *are associated with advanced glycation end products (AGEs) via hypertrophy and osteogenic differentiation. Histological analyses of human IVDs from several degeneration stages revealed areas of ectopic calcification within the nucleus pulposus and at the cartilage endplate. These ectopic calcifications were associated with cells positive for the AGE methylglyoxal-hydroimidazolone-1 (MG-H1). MG-H1 was also co-localized with Collagen 10 (COL10) and Osteopontin (OPN) suggesting osteogenic differentiation. Bovine nucleus pulposus and cartilaginous endplate cells in cell culture demonstrated that 200 mg/mL AGEs in low-glucose media increased ectopic calcifications after 4 d in culture and significantly increased COL10 and OPN expression. The receptor for AGE (RAGE) was involved in this differentiation process since its inhibition reduced COL10 and OPN expression. We conclude that AGE accumulation is associated with endochondral ossification in IVDs and likely acts via the AGE/RAGE axis to induce hypertrophy and osteogenic differentiation in IVD cells. We postulate that this ectopic calcification may play an important role in accelerated IVD degeneration including the initiation of structural defects. Since orally administered AGE and RAGE inhibitors are available, future investigations on AGE/RAGE and endochondral ossification may be a promising direction for developing a non-invasive treatment against the progression of IVD degeneration.*

This report makes me wonder, how long will it take until the FDA or the USDA to wake up and realize that what they're recommending everyone eat is actually what's making everyone sick. Then I think about who controls the FDA and the USDA, it somehow nullifies my curiosity, I know who is responsible. A multinational chemical company intent on bolstering their profits at whatever cost, regardless of what may be brought about their actions.

It's when those actions bolster the profits of another related industry that I get bothered. When I see people conned into consuming foods that make them sicker every day, I get a little upset. When I see this, I see my mother dying because she bought into this ruse herself. This makes this ruse the most dangerous con game ever to hit mankind.

The following report submitted Mar 2, 2009, details the beginning of glycation from the fundamental elements of glucose, glyoxal and methylglyoxal, and their roles in aging and disease;

- **Protein and nucleotide damage by glyoxal and methylglyoxal in physiological systems - role in aging and disease**

Glyoxal and methylglyoxal are potent glycating agents. Glycation of proteins is a complex series of parallel and sequential reactions collectively called the Maillard reaction. It occurs in all tissues and body fluids. Early stage reactions in glycation of protein by glucose lead to the formation of fructose-lysine (FL) and N-terminal amino acid residue-derived fructosamines. Later stage reactions form stable end-stage adducts called advanced glycation endproducts (AGEs). FL degrades slowly to form AGEs – and also glyoxal and methylglyoxal. In contrast, glyoxal and methylglyoxal react with proteins to form AGE residues directly and relatively rapidly.

Glycation by glyoxal and methylglyoxal, and the related influence of Glo1 are now emerging as playing a critical role in aging and disease processes – vascular complications associated with diabetes renal failure, Alzheimer's disease, and tumorigenesis and multidrug resistance in cancer chemotherapy. They may also have roles in pathologic anxiety, autism, obesity and other disorders.

Again, this is just one of 804 return reports from a search of Lymphoma and glycation. To think that one has nothing to do with the other is what the FDA and the USDA seem to be doing in the continued recommendations to eat the food that does the glycating. If you were to tell me that the influence of Monsanto's execs in the offices and agencies had nothing to do with these decisions to alert the public about the dangers in what they're eating, I'd have to tell you that you are completely misinformed. Can I sell you some ocean front property in Kansas?

Does this mean that you're stupid? Absolutely not. It just means that you've been duped like everyone else. It's really easy to do. All you have to do is taste the food. One taste and you're hooked. Since it doesn't kill you immediately, it's assumed safe. This assumption is what's killing America and the rest of the world. This is the most deadly assumption to make, bread is safe to eat. Bread nowadays is deadly...very deadly

When I searched glycation and asthma, it returned 45 studies showing the influence that glycation has on asthma. The first one explains how more severe asthma can be characterized by clustering of AGEs;

- **A Systemic Inflammatory Endotype of Asthma With More Severe Disease Identified by Unbiased Clustering of the Serum Cytokine Profile.**

Asthma is considered as a clinical and molecularly heterogeneous disorder. Systemic inflammation is suggested to play an important role in a group of asthma patients. We hypothesized that there is a subgroup of patients with asthma characterized by systemic inflammation. In this study, we aimed to discriminate asthma subtypes based on circulating biomarkers and to determine whether a systemic inflammatory endotype of asthma could be identified. In the present cross-sectional study, 50 patients with untreated asthma were prospectively recruited from a single academic outpatient clinic, and characterized with respect to clinical, functional, and inflammatory parameters. The expression profiles of 20 serum cytokines were assessed by anti-human cytokine antibody array. Then, hierarchical clustering analysis was performed based on the principal component analysis (PCA)-transformed data to classify the clinical groups. PCA showed that 6 independent components accounted for 80.113% of the variance, and PCA-based hierarchical clustering identified 3 endotypes. One of the endotypes was evidenced by elevated systemic inflammation markers such as leptin, vascular endothelial growth factor (VEGF), and reduced levels of soluble receptor for advanced glycation end products (sRAGE), an anti-inflammatory molecule. More female patients were included, with higher circulating neutrophil counts and more severe symptoms. In conclusion, we identified an endotype of asthma characterized by systemic inflammation and severe symptoms. Increased levels of VEGF, leptin and decreased level of sRAGE may contribute to the systemic inflammation of this asthma endotype.

With inflammation being a major influence on asthma, would it make sense to control the inflammation first and foremost?

This report from Oct 16, 2015, details how high fructose corn syrup is associated with chronic bronchitis;

- **Intake of high fructose corn syrup sweetened soft drinks is associated with prevalent chronic bronchitis in U.S. Adults, ages 20-55 y.**

High fructose corn syrup (HFCS) sweetened soft drink intake has been linked with asthma in US high-schoolers. Intake of beverages with excess free fructose (EFF), including apple juice, and HFCS sweetened fruit drinks and soft drinks, has been associated with asthma in children. One hypothesis for this association is that underlying fructose malabsorption and fructose reactivity in the GI may contribute to in situ formations of enFruAGEs. EnFruAGEs may be an overlooked source of advanced glycation end-products (AGE) that contribute to lung disease. AGE/ RAGEs are elevated in COPD lungs. EFF intake has increased in recent decades, and intakes may exceed dosages associated with adult fructose malabsorption in subsets of the population. Intestinal dysfunction has been shown to be elevated in COPD patients. The objective of this study was to investigate the association between HFCS sweetened soft drink intake and chronic bronchitis (CB), a common manifestation of COPD, in adults.

HFCS sweetened soft drink intake is correlated with chronic bronchitis in US adults aged 20-55 y, after adjusting for covariates, including smoking. Results support the hypothesis that underlying fructose malabsorption and fructose reactivity in the GI may contribute to chronic bronchitis, perhaps through in situ formations of enFruAGEs, which may contribute to lung disease. Longitudinal and biochemical research is needed to confirm and clarify the mechanisms involved.

The next report I looked at was from Nov 10, 2016, and it displays the extent this industry will go to, to simply allow this addiction to killing as many people as it possibly can, by it to continue. Its purpose is to show the benefits of Bazedoxifene, a new drug being tested for reducing apoptosis and oxidative stress when all they have to do is to recommend the cessation of the consumption of grains and sugar that leads to the glycation that is responsible for all these diseases. They're not interested in arresting it or abating it. Their sole interest is to expand its influence, to addict more and more people. This appears to be done solely to increase the profits of the pharmaceutical industry. It explains the benefits of a new drug that the industry wants to impose upon the people, probably in the guise of helping the people;

- **Bazedoxifene Ameliorates Homocysteine-Induced Apoptosis and Accumulation of Advanced Glycation End Products by Reducing Oxidative Stress in MC3T3-E1 Cells.**

Abstract

Elevated plasma homocysteine (Hcy) level increases the risk of osteoporotic fracture by deteriorating bone quality. However, little is known about the effects of Hcy on osteoblast and collagen cross-links. This study aimed to investigate whether Hcy induces apoptosis of osteoblastic MC3T3-E1 cells as well as affects enzymatic and nonenzymatic collagen cross-links and to determine the effects of bazedoxifene, a selective estrogen receptor modulator, on the Hcy-induced apoptosis and deterioration of collagen cross-links in the cells. Hcy treatments (300 µM, 3 mM, and 10 mM) increased intracellular reactive oxygen species (ROS) production in a dose-dependent manner. Propidium iodide staining showed that 3 and 10 mM Hcy induced apoptosis of MC3T3-E1 cells. Moreover, the activities of caspases-8, 9, and 3 were increased by 3 mM Hcy. The detrimental effects of 3 mM Hcy on apoptosis and ROS production were partly reversed by bazedoxifene and 17β estradiol. In addition, real-time PCR, immunostaining and Western blot showed that 300 µM Hcy decreased the expression of lysyl oxidase (Lox). Furthermore, 300 µM Hcy increased extracellular accumulation of pentosidine, an advanced glycation end product. Treatment with bazedoxifene ameliorated Hcy-induced suppression of Lox expression and increase in pentosidine accumulation. These findings suggest that high-dose Hcy induces apoptosis of osteoblasts by increasing oxidative stress, and low-dose Hcy decreases enzymatic collagen cross-links and increases pentosidine accumulation, resulting in the deterioration of bone quality. Bazedoxifene treatment effectively prevents the Hcy-induced detrimental reactions of osteoblasts. Thus, bazedoxifene may be a potential therapeutic drug for preventing Hcy-induced bone fragility.

Even though we've had an idea of the damage of glycation and what causes it for over 30 years, This industry is still concentrating on making new drugs. Drugs always have side effects that lead to more drugs, yet this is this industry's modus operandi. They don't know how to operate otherwise. It's the ties to the grains industry that I object to and the power we've given to these industries, simply to allow the public to continue to feed their addiction. You might as well tell us to stand in front of a racing bus or semi. You're basically selling us the same thing, future time in the hospital;

Bazedoxifene Ameliorates Homocysteine-Induced Apoptosis and Accumulation of Advanced Glycation End Products by Reducing Oxidative Stress in MC3T3-E1 Cells.

Abstract

Elevated plasma homocysteine (Hcy) level increases the risk of osteoporotic fracture by deteriorating bone quality. However, little is known about the effects of Hcy on osteoblast and collagen cross-links. This study aimed to investigate whether Hcy induces apoptosis of osteoblastic MC3T3-E1 cells as well as affects enzymatic and nonenzymatic collagen cross-links and to determine the effects of bazedoxifene, a selective estrogen receptor modulator, on the Hcy-induced apoptosis and deterioration of collagen cross-links in the cells. Hcy treatments (300 µM, 3 mM, and 10 mM) increased intracellular reactive oxygen species (ROS) production in a dose-dependent manner. Propidium iodide staining showed that 3 and 10 mM Hcy induced apoptosis of MC3T3-E1 cells. Moreover, the activities of caspases-8, 9, and 3 were increased by 3 mM Hcy. The detrimental effects of 3 mM Hcy on apoptosis and ROS production were partly reversed by bazedoxifene and 17β estradiol. In addition, real-time PCR, immunostaining and Western blot showed that 300 µM Hcy decreased the expression of lysyl oxidase (Lox). Furthermore, 300 µM Hcy increased extracellular accumulation of pentosidine, an advanced glycation end product. Treatment with bazedoxifene ameliorated Hcy-induced suppression of Lox expression and increase in pentosidine accumulation. These findings suggest that high-dose Hcy induces apoptosis of osteoblasts by increasing oxidative stress, and low-dose Hcy decreases enzymatic collagen cross-links and increases pentosidine accumulation, resulting in the deterioration of bone quality. Bazedoxifene treatment effectively prevents the Hcy-induced detrimental reactions of osteoblasts. Thus, bazedoxifene may be a potential therapeutic drug for preventing Hcy-induced bone fragility.

This displays the true despair of this problem, an industry more intent on driving profits than healing the people they affect. Their only interest is in making more drugs to allow the continuation of an addiction that's putting more people in the hospital than any other one thing. To me, that is the definition of criminal behavior. This is a clear indication of legal extortion....and we allow it to continue, just to feed our addiction.

This next report dated Oct 18, 2016, shows the influence of Metformin on the AGE population in our blood. It turns out to be another way to get you to take more drugs, as this drug encourages increased levels of CML (another AGE).

- **Plasma Levels of Pentosidine, Carboxymethyl-Lysine, Soluble Receptor for Advanced Glycation End Products, and Metabolic Syndrome: The Metformin Effect.**

Abstract

Metabolic syndrome (Mets) is considered one of the most important public health problems. Several and controversial studies showed that the role of advanced glycation end products (AGEs) and their receptor in the development of metabolic syndrome and therapeutic pathways is still unsolved. We have investigated whether plasma pentosidine, carboxymethyl-lysine (CML), and soluble receptor for advanced glycation end products (sRAGE) levels were increased in patients with Mets and the effect of metformin in plasma levels of pentosidine, CML, and sRAGE. 80 control subjects and 86 patients were included in this study. Pentosidine, CML, and sRAGE were measured in plasma by enzyme-linked immunosorbent assay (ELISA). Plasma pentosidine, CML, and sRAGE levels were significantly increased in patients compared to control subjects (P < 0.001, P < 0.001, and P = 0.014, resp.). Plasma levels of pentosidine were significantly decreased in patients who received metformin compared to untreated patients (P = 0.01). However, there was no significant difference between patients treated with metformin and untreated patients in plasma CML levels. Plasma levels of sRAGE were significantly increased in patients who received metformin and ACE inhibitors (P < 0.001 and P = 0.002, resp.). However, in a multiple stepwise regression analysis, pentosidine, sRAGE, and drugs treatments were not independently associated. Patients with metabolic syndrome showed increased levels of AGEs such as pentosidine and CML. Metformin treatment showed a decreased level of pentosidine but not of CML. Therapeutic pathways of AGEs development should be taken into account and further experimental and in vitro studies merit for advanced research.

The purpose of this study was to look at Metformin's effect on two different AGEs, pentosidine and CML. Again the emphasis is on finding ways to keep the glycating substances in the diet and offering treatment only, not in finding a cure. That would involve removing the glycating substances from the diet and that would hurt the grain industry. Their treatment though involves the continuation of their prescribed drug regimen. This is why they pay the prettiest reps to sell their drugs to all the doctors who prescribe them.

Below is evidence that the destruction of glycation starts before you were ever born, thanks to your mother's glucose ingestion. This is where your addiction began. Do you think if she knew how much harm she was inflicting, she would do it again? That might depend on her addiction. From the study report itself, dated Nov 2016;

- **High-fructose diet in pregnancy leads to fetal programming of hypertension, insulin resistance, and obesity in adult offspring.**

Abstract

BACKGROUND:

Consumption of fructose-rich diets in the United States is on the rise and thought to be associated with obesity and cardiometabolic diseases.

OBJECTIVE:

We sought to determine the effects of antenatal exposure to high-fructose diet on offspring's development of metabolic syndrome-like phenotype and other cardiovascular disease risk factors later in life.

STUDY DESIGN:

Pregnant C57BL/6J dams were randomly allocated to fructose solution (10% wt/vol, n = 10) or water (n = 10) as the only drinking fluid from day 1 of pregnancy until delivery. After weaning, pups were started on regular chow and evaluated at 1 year of life. We measured percent visceral adipose tissue and liver fat infiltrates using computed tomography, and blood pressure using CODA noninvasive monitor. Intraperitoneal glucose tolerance testing with corresponding insulin concentrations was obtained. Serum concentrations of glucose, insulin, triglycerides, total cholesterol, leptin, and adiponectin were measured in duplicate using standardized assays. Fasting homeostatic model assessment was also calculated to assess insulin resistance. P values <.05 were considered statistically significant.

RESULTS:

Maternal weight, pup number, and average weight at birth were similar between the 2 groups. Male and female fructose group offspring had higher peak glucose and area under the intraperitoneal glucose tolerance testing curve compared with control, and higher mean arterial pressure compared to control. Female fructose group offspring were heavier and had higher percent visceral adipose tissue, liver fat infiltrates, homeostatic model assessment of insulin resistance scores, insulin area under the intraperitoneal glucose tolerance testing curve, and serum concentrations of leptin, and lower concentrations of adiponectin compared to female control offspring. No significant differences in these parameters were noted in male offspring. Serum concentrations of triglycerides or total cholesterol were not different between the 2 groups for either gender.

CONCLUSION:

Maternal intake of high fructose leads to fetal programming of adult obesity, hypertension, and metabolic dysfunction, all risk factors for cardiovascular disease. This fetal programming is more pronounced in female offspring. Limiting intake of high fructose-enriched diets in pregnancy may have a significant impact on long-term health.

Are these enough reports to prove what directly influences diabetes? After reading this can you see the logic in controlling your diabetes by controlling your carb intake? Where are the warnings from the FDA and the USDA? Don't they care about what they're recommending? Don't they understand because of their recommendations, they send millions of Moms and Dads, sisters, and brothers, husbands and wives to their slow, expensive, painful deaths?

- **Monocyte Chemotactic Protein-1, Fractalkine, and Receptor for Advanced Glycation End Products in Different Pathological**

Types of Lupus Nephritis and Their Value in Different Treatment Prognoses.

BACKGROUND:

Early diagnosis is important for the outcome of lupus nephritis (LN). However, the pathological type of lupus nephritis closely related to the clinical manifestations; therefore, the treatment of lupus nephritis depends on the different pathological types.

OBJECTIVE:

To assess the level of monocyte chemotactic protein (MCP-1), fractalkine (Fkn), and receptor for advanced glycation end product (RAGE) in different pathological types of lupus nephritis and to explore the value of these biomarkers for predicting the prognosis of lupus nephritis.

METHODS:

Patients included in this study were assessed using renal biopsy. Class III and class IV were defined as the proliferative group, class V as a non-proliferative group, and class V+III and class V+IV as the mixed group. During the follow-up, 40 of 178 enrolled patients had a poor response to the standard immunosuppressant therapy. The level of markers in the different response groups was tested.

RESULTS:

The levels of urine and serum MCP-1, urine and serum fractalkine, and serum RAGE were higher in the proliferative group, and lower in the non-proliferative group, and this difference was significant. The levels of urine and serum MCP-1 and serum RAGE were lower in the poor response group, and these differences were also significant. The relationship between urine MCP-1 and urine and serum fractalkine with the systemic lupus erythematosus disease activity index was evaluated.

CONCLUSION:

The concentration of cytokines MCP-1, fractalkine, and RAGE may be correlated with different pathology type of lupus nephritis. Urine and serum MCP-1 and serum RAGE may help in predicting the prognosis prior to standard immunosuppressant therapy.

Do you have Lupus? Were you told not to eat your bagels for breakfast? If you weren't, then it's probably because someone needed you back for treatment.

This following report dated

- **HMGB1 Promotes Systemic Lupus Erythematosus by Enhancing Macrophage Inflammatory Response.**

Background/Purpose: HMGB1, which may act as a proinflammatory mediator, has been proposed to contribute to the pathogenesis of multiple chronic inflammatories and autoimmune diseases including systemic lupus erythematosus (SLE); however, the precise mechanism of HMGB1 in the pathogenic process of SLE remains obscure.

Method: The expression of HMGB1 was measured by ELISA and western blot. The ELISA was also applied to detect proinflammatory cytokines levels. Furthermore, nephritic pathology was evaluated by H&E staining of renal tissues. Results: In this study, we found that HMGB1 levels were significantly increased and correlated with SLE disease activity in both clinical patients and a murine model. Furthermore, gain- and loss-of-function analysis showed that HMGB1 exacerbated the severity of SLE. Of note, the HMGB1 levels were found to be associated with the levels of proinflammatory cytokines such as TNF-α and IL-6 in SLE patients. Further study demonstrated that increased HMGB1 expression deteriorated the severity of SLE via enhancing macrophage inflammatory response. Moreover, we found that receptor of advanced glycation end products played a critical role in HMGB1-mediated macrophage inflammatory response.

Conclusion: These findings suggested that HMGB1 might be a risk factor for SLE, and manipulation of HMGB1 signaling might provide a therapeutic strategy for SLE.

With this kind of evidence, do you think this might suggest that a ketogenic diet would be healthier?

Another study proving the role of glycation in the pathogenesis of arthritis proves once again how inflammation is the result of glycation, something you have control over:

- **The potential role of advanced glycation end products (AGEs) and soluble receptors for AGEs (sRAGE) in the pathogenesis of adult-onset Still's disease.**

BACKGROUND:

Accumulating evidence has demonstrated a pathogenic role of advanced glycation end products (AGEs) and receptors for AGEs (RAGE) in inflammation. Soluble RAGE (sRAGE), with the same ligand-binding capacity as full-length RAGE, acts as a "decoy" receptor. However, there has been scanty data regarding AGEs and sRAGE in adult-onset Still's disease (AOSD). This study aimed to investigate AGEs and sRAGE levels in AOSD patients and examine their association with clinical characteristics.

METHODS:

Using ELISA, plasma levels of AGEs and sRAGE were determined in 52 AOSD patients, 36 systemic lupus erythematosus(SLE) patients and 16 healthy controls(HC). Their associations with activity parameters and disease courses were evaluated.

RESULTS:

Significantly higher median levels of AGEs were observed in active AOSD patients (16.75 pg/ml) and active SLE patients (14.80 pg/ml) than those in

HC (9.80 pg/ml, both p < 0.001). AGEs levels were positively correlated with activity scores (r = 0.836, p < 0.001), ferritin levels (r = 0.372, p < 0.05) and CRP levels (r = 0.396, p < 0.005) in AOSD patients. Conversely, significantly lower median levels of sRAGE were observed in active AOSD patients (632.2 pg/ml) and active SLE patients (771.6 pg/ml) compared with HC (1051.7 pg/ml, both p < 0.001). Plasma sRAGE levels were negatively correlated with AOSD activity scores (r = -0.320, p < 0.05). In comparison to AOSD patients with monocyclic pattern, significantly higher AGEs levels were observed in those with polycyclic or chronic articular pattern. With treatment, AGEs levels declined while sRAGE levels increased in parallel with the decrease in disease activity.

CONCLUSION:

The elevation of AGEs levels with concomitant decreased sRAGE levels in active AOSD patients, suggests their pathogenic role in AOSD.

Juvenile arthritis is shown in this study to be the product of glycation, again something you have control over by what goes into your body for food. If you or your child suffers from this, your only cure is to stop the glycation. The older you are, the less you can reverse. But if you're young enough, you may be able to reverse a majority of it.

- **The presence of high mobility group box-1 and soluble receptor for advanced glycation end-products in juvenile idiopathic arthritis and juvenile systemic lupus erythematosus.**

Background

The involvement of high mobility group box-1 (HMGB1) in various inflammatory and autoimmune diseases has been documented but clinical trials on the contribution of this pro-inflammatory alarmin in children with juvenile idiopathic arthritis (JIA) and systemic lupus erythematosus (SLE) are basically absent. To address the presence of HMGB1 and a soluble receptor for advanced glycation end products (sRAGE) in different subtypes of JIA and additionally in children with SLE, we enrolled a consecutive sample of children harvested peripheral blood as well as synovial fluids (SF) at diagnosis and correlated it with ordinary acute-phase reactants and clinical markers.

Methods

Serum and synovial fluids levels of HMGB1 and sRAGE in a total of 144 children (97 with JIA, 19 with SLE and 27 healthy controls) were determined by ELISA.

Results

The children with JIA and those with SLE were characterized by significantly higher serum levels of HMGB1 and significantly lower sRAGE levels compared to the healthy controls. A positive correlation between serum HMGB1 and ESR, CRP, α2 globulin was found while serum sRAGE levels were inversely correlated with the same inflammatory markers in children with JIA. Additionally, high level of serum HMGB1 was related to hepatosplenomegaly or serositis in systemic-onset JIA.

Conclusion

The inverse relationship of the HMGB1 and its soluble receptor RAGE in the blood and SF indicates that inflammation triggered by alarmins may play a role in the pathogenesis of JIA as well as SLE. HMGB1 may serve as an inflammatory marker and a potential target of biological therapy in these patients. Further studies need to show whether the determination of HMGB1 levels in patients with JIA can be a useful guideline for detecting disease activity.

What's important is that you stop the introduction of glucose as soon as possible to arrest the glycation. The secret to this cure is an end to all glycation. The magic of this cure is the end of the hunger cycle and pain. (I've noticed that they go together.)

These are free reports that are available to everyone. All you have to do is search for them at the National Library of Medicine in the National Institute of Health. There are literally 100s of thousands of reports on the effects of glycation that remain hidden in the PubMed and PMC databases except to the few who look through them. The only ones looking through this database are the drug companies looking for more ways to make money. Nobody is looking to warn anyone of the dangers of this food.

My question is why? The answer I get is, "there's no money in it". That's why I said in my first book, it would be a shame if profits and money weren't the primary motivating factors in our society, but they are, and we have to live with it. That's why I choose not to buy into it. It's the same choice you have.

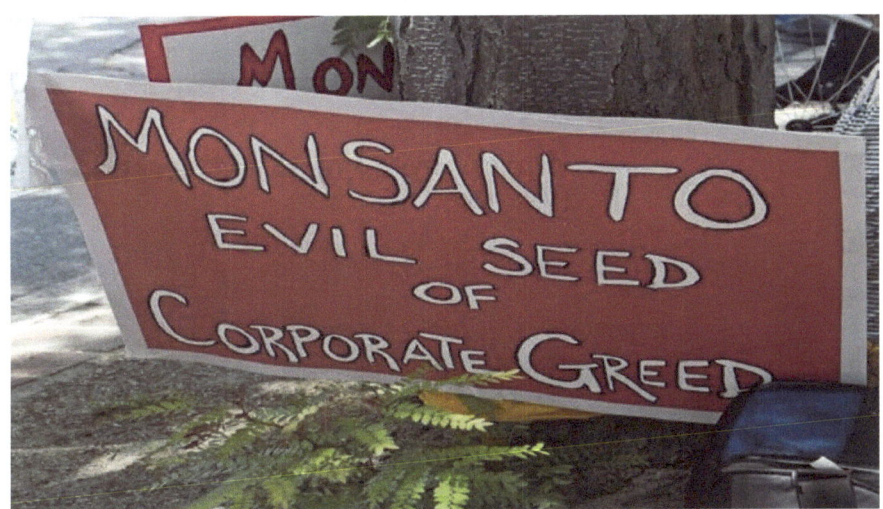

CHAPTER 8

UNDERSTANDING THE REAL REASON WHY WE FIGHT

I can still remember it today. It was the absolute best feeling that I've ever had. I can remember exactly how I thought, what time of day it was, the room we were in. My memory of this special event is locked in my mind, forever. I thought this is so good, how can anyone fall out of love after this. I remember uttering that same feeling and hearing, "I wouldn't know. I love you too." I said again, but this time with more conviction, "I love you so much...I don't know how I could ever stop loving you."

That was the day we lost our cherries. I saw the spot on the sheets after we finished and asked her what it was, not knowing. When I did realize what it was, I felt ashamed for not knowing, then I fell deeper in love. She and I had shared something physically sacred that you experience only once in your life. When I realized what she had given up to secure my love, I relinquished my love to her without reservation or hesitation. I knew at that moment that she was my soul mate. I couldn't imagine being with anyone else or anything coming between us. I also couldn't realize what would eventually drive a wedge between us, to drive us apart.

Looking back on it now, I know exactly what it was that drove us apart. It was my pride. She was smarter than I and due to that fact, I had trouble acknowledging her superior intellect. I wasn't used to not always being "right". Because she was smarter than I, she had this habit of being right more often than I and that was tough for me to accept. I wish now that I could have worked a little harder at understanding. I've never stopped loving her and never will. She is still my soul mate, except she's with someone else because of my behavior.

Looking back on our relationship, it was rocky. I think I know why that was. I think it was because of our carbohydrate diet and the hunger cycles it put us through. I didn't know it at that time, but the hunger was the driving force behind every other cycle I went through. I was raised on bread, mostly because my mother loved it and she loved it immensely. At that time, in the fifties, bread wasn't the nasty stuff that it is now. Then it was the staff of life. Now, it's the staff of death. As I was raised on bread, I had a more active hunger cycle and because of this hunger cycle, I found myself in more trouble than most other kids my age and I was always in trouble of some sort, usually due to the fact that I couldn't control my emotions. Emotions are always the first to go on a hunger cycle. This is due to the fact that they're controlled by your hormones which are controlled by your diet. This was something it took me 60 years to learn. I wish now that I knew then what I know now, but I couldn't. I was locked into an addiction that kept me from seeing any danger signs except that I needed to make some changes.

There was an industry intent on not allowing us to know. That same industry had intentions of using our love of bread for their benefit, seeing an opportunity to make money out of an addiction that we grew into. We've had this affliction all of our lives. We were born into it as it starts before we're born, due to the consumption of it by our mothers who couldn't break away from it. That's because they're born into it. We're all born into it. It's the nature of how this grain has shaped our civilization.

It's shaped our civilization through its hunger cycle which has also forced us to reap the reward of that cycle. Like all cycles, it has its ups and downs and this is what condemns us to the karma we've created through our hunger cycles. When we're hungry, we act with less forethought and concern for long-term consequences of our actions. This doesn't allow us to see all of those manifestations, prior to our committing them. We only see the ones we want to see and this is where we get into trouble. Because of our clouded judgment, we not open to all possibilities or consequences of those possibilities and this is why our karma comes back to bite us. Too often that karma comes back in the form of terrorism when our hasty decisions are international and affect other people and nationalities. This turns the war on terrorism into a war on sugar and grains, our real nemeses.

Due to the fact that this grain has shaped our history so much, it's influenced the usurping of more territory than any other one reason. Capturing land that grew this important food meant that the conqueror could control the people that this grain fed. That meant security for the owner of such land. It was the wealth that brought this security that drove this kind of behavior, but it was the underlying hunger that drove the desire for security. This is a natural reaction to the hormonal imbalance that the hunger cycle brings with it everywhere it goes. This is due to the influence that sugar and glucose have on those hormones. They're devastating, to say the least, and they keep your hormones from being under your own control. Because of that, your hormones are under the control of what you're eating. Your diet of carbohydrates makes certain of this.

In my opinion, it's also what leads to all abhorrent behavior that in my eyes is evil. Because this behavior is driven by fear and since fear is what drives all evil, it's my opinion that this food can be considered a driver of evil. It didn't use to be like that, but it is now, especially with glyphosate that's been dumped, on these crops. Tons of the enzyme inhibiting weed killer is changing our hormonal balance to the point where it's not safe to eat bread anymore. Nor is it safe to eat corn, oats or any grain, for that matter, even sugar. They all get desiccated before harvest and this is where the danger is, in the desiccating of the crop for higher-yielding harvest. This one action alone ensures that we get enough glyphosate into our diets to ensure our compliance into the glucose ruse of a never-ending drug cycle that can only end in a premature death.

All grains (including sugar) are soaked in so much glyphosate that they can't help but rearrange your hormones and ultimately, health. This is why so many people are dying today from all modern disease that exists. This glyphosate actually ramps up the glycation that's responsible for these diseases and disorders and the general public isn't aware of this. They don't know what's really behind these pandemics of obesity and diabetes, cardiovascular and heart diseases as well as all cancers and dementias. They just know that what tastes good and unfortunately, that just happens to be the same thing that does all the damage. All this damage is due to the glycation that this food instigates and the fact that the glycation has been magnified by the glyphosate that it's been drenched in. This is a recipe for disaster for the health of the public. It's also a recipe for profit for;

1. the seed companies that provide the GMO seed,
2. the chemical industry that provides the glyphosate herbicide
3. pharmaceutical industries that treat you for your pain.

This profit comes from your pockets and your health. Is your addiction worth it? So, what can you do, to stay away from this glycating sugar in your diet? Nothing except to give it up...forever. This is the only way you can be free of its addiction, as it has addicted us unwittingly. It did this as soon as we were able to eat it. When one compares the ancient civilizations and their aggressive nature, the most aggressive civilizations were the ones under the influence of wheat and grains more than anything else. These crops became staples in our diet, where they used to only be eaten small amounts as it took a long time to gather it up, in order to eat it.

The Celtic empire that never had a territory, shows this clearly. The Celts were a tall people. this is due to the protein in the wheat, amylopectin. It enabled the people who ate this einkorn wheat to grow taller and more muscular. What it did underneath the surface was completely hidden until just recently when AGEs were discovered and the real destruction of this kind of diet presented itself. That's in the glycation that these grains create.

The domestication of the grain into crops to feed the masses gave this food, power over the masses and landowners power to control that power. Landowners knew this and that's why they invaded fertile lands first. It was this land that could provide them with enough food to feed their armies. This was the perfect food to feed an army, as you could more easily control this army by controlling their hunger. Powerful warlords knew that whoever controlled the food, controlled the people.

What they didn't know, it was their own hunger that influenced this behavior and that it was the influence of their diets that influenced their hunger. That's something I didn't know until just recently. It took removing them from my diet to fully understand it, but it's plain as day, now that I'm outside of the addiction. One can seldom see an addiction when they're stuck in it and this is the inherent danger in this grain. It's always been addictive, ever since we've been eating it. It always will be and since we've eaten this food all of our lives, as we ate it when we're infants, that addicts us unwittingly and forever, unless we're aware of it wiles, its dangers, and it's addictive nature.

Any substance that affects your hormones like sugar and grains do, is going to be addictive. Alcohol proves this. So does heroin and every other drug. But then so does gambling and all risk-taking, for that fact, because it's driven by a cycle of greed, which is driven by the hunger cycle. This is why a contend that all terrorism is driven by a hunger cycle which is driven by sugar and carbs. This is also why I contend that all wars were and are ultimately driven by a hunger cycle because a power grab is a manifestation of a hunger cycle. It's the idea of security that drives someone to gain more power. It's this idea of security that's prompted by the hunger cycle. Who wants to go hungry?

Because I've broken my hunger cycle by breaking my addiction, I can see this clearly, right now. You could easier understand this concept if you can break your hunger cycle also.

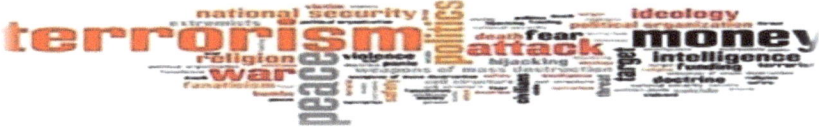

THE BEST WAY TO FIGHT HUNGER FIGHTS TERRORISM AS WELL

You know better than I do that hunger pervades our society. Everybody experiences hunger every day. Some people experience hunger all day all night long. At least it's thought so. Actually, those who go without food don't often experience hunger except for the ones who haven't broken the cycle of hunger. This is a cycle that controls hunger a few hours at a time at a time. This is also an addiction. This is your addiction to glucose. It works by playing with your hormones every time your blood glucose levels change. When you eat carbs your glucose levels are altered, it's this alteration of your blood glucose levels that alter the reaction of your hormones. It's those changes in your hormones that affect your behavior and makes you act in the manner you do. It's those changes in hormones that also affect your hunger cycles. I call it the *Glucose Ruse*. It's only deadly to those who buy into it. I won't because I won't pay for terrorism.

This is simple. At least, to me, it's simple. Actually, this may be the easiest and simplest cure for hunger that exists today. If you think it's time for a cure for hunger, I've got the solution for the world; to best fight hunger, you need to stop the hunger cycle. You need to do this not by feeding starving people bags of flour and corn to eat, but by giving them education about nutrition and diet to get them off of the flour and corn diet. That is what makes them hungry and dependent on the grains for their diet. They will remain dependent until they either quit eating the grains or die. The death part always comes prematurely, always. This is the addiction part of the cycle.

Since you can live better without carbs (I'm proving that), your body does not need them. That is the definition of addiction, the body requiring something it doesn't need and manifesting discomfort when it's not available for the affected to use. This is the same as what an alcoholic goes through when they can't get a drink. It's what cigarette smokers feel when they need a smoke. It's a need that has to be satisfied, but it can only be satisfied in your mind, where your hormones affect your emotions. They affect your emotions in your mind, more than anywhere else. This is your instruction center for the body, for what happens in the body and how you react to whatever stimuli affect the body.

How Sugar Creates Terrorism

Your emotions should remain in your control, not in the control of what you eat. When you allow that to happen, you're allowing the industry that controls what you eat, to control how you feel and what you do, by controlling your emotions. This is a cycle. It's a cycle of dependence. It's a cycle of dependence on the grain industry. Not the beef industry or dairy industry, simply the grain industry and its manufacturers and processors. It's this industry that's responsible for all glycation that occurs in your blood. It's this industry that's responsible for your hunger cycles and that put's responsibility on them for your changes in emotions and behavior. It can also give them some responsibility for the terrorism that exists in the world today as it's controlled by the amount of anger and hate that's expressed which in turn is controlled by what controls the hate and anger and that's a glucose diet. It's this diet, that's responsible for your emotional changes. by changing your hormones. This diet creates this hunger cycle that all who are living on it can expect to live with. Hunger is the cost of a diet of carbohydrates. It's that simple.

It's not only a cycle of hunger, it's a cycle of addiction. Every addict has to feed their addiction. When you feel hungry, what do you hunger for? What is the first thing you want to eat or drink? That tells you where your addiction lies. I know what you're thinking right now, how can hunger to eat be an addiction? That's the first question I'm asked, whenever I call this an addiction.

This is how addictions work, they force your body to want something that it really doesn't need. It creates discomfort in the body until that need is met. When that need is met, comfort takes place and damage internally begins. While your emotions are being controlled by your glucose infusion and making you feel comfortable, the glucose from the sugar and carbs is busy, very busy glycating whatever cholesterol or protein the glucose can find. Even though it's not the glycation the creates the hunger, (the hunger comes from hormone imbalance, but then, so does the pain, discomfort, irritability and general malaise that these grains bring), the glycation is now a more clarified manifestation of the real damage that takes place, every time this substance is eaten. (Thanks to Dr. Davis, Dr. Perlmutter, Dr. Volek, PubMed, and PMC.)

Those grains not only increase hunger, but they're the prime agents behind all modern diseases caused by the creation of glycation in the blood. That's exactly what these foods do. How they do it, right now, isn't important. What's important is that these foods, in the manner in which they are digested, not only create the glycation but they create hunger as well. It's this hunger they create that makes them addictive and dangerous to the point of deadly.

It has to do with the fluctuation of your hormones due to your diet of grains. Once grains are ground, they lose their fiber. This is important because it's the fiber that slows down the breakdown of the sugars in the grains that influence your blood glucose. The slower those sugars are introduced into your system, the slower they raise your blood glucose. Most diabetics know this, as it's the quick rise in blood glucose that is responsible for the glycation and the release of hormones that actually work to increase your hunger.

Leptin which is supposed to keep you from being hungry is actually increased to the point where it does little good for your body anymore. There's so much of it in your body that you don't recognize what you've already eaten and this is what's dangerous. It's this leptin resistance that makes you hungry.

This is what drives the hunger cycle and most all restaurants know this. (This is why they give you bread as soon as they seat you.) This is what makes everyone hungry. My theory is to eliminate this cycle, and to do that, means changing the equation, the equation of digestion. The best way to change that equation is to changes the factors of the equation, in this case, one factor. All you have to do to cure hunger and glycation is to remove that which creates hunger and glycation, carbohydrates from the equation and thus the diet. The solution is that simple. Maybe not easy, but simple.

When one considers the fact that the primary driver of hunger is a carbohydrate diet, it's easy to see that the solution for hunger is to eliminate the cycle of hunger by changing the diet. Taking carbohydrates out of the diet removes the hunger factor and thus the hunger cycle. Anyone doubting this can go on the diet that I've been on for three years and they'll know this to be true. Three years on the diet that I've been on will not only convince anyone of this concept, it will also improve their health in unimaginable ways. The last time I got hungry was 3 yrs 3 months ago. That was when I broke my addiction to glucose. Others who are on this diet will tell you the same thing, they don't get hungry and the reason they don't get hungry is that they don't have the glucose going through their systems to create the hunger cycle.

Because this is an addiction, those who still eat carbs, can't see it. You have to break the addiction to know this. That's the way it is with any addiction, you can't see it while you're in it. Yet, almost everyone knows that sugar is addictive. I think because nobody wants to equate that sugar with carbs, they don't want to fully grasp that the carbs they were told they need, is sugar. Carbs, something you were told you had to have, breaks down to the exact same thing as sugar, and that's glucose, and glucose glycates and makes you hungry.

Yet, they're still telling everyone to eat whole grains, as though they're healthy. It's always been spoken of in that manner because it justified our need for it. That, my friends, is the definition of dependency and I think you know what that deals with when the dependency deals with a substance. This dependency has infiltrated the agencies that are supposed to regulate it, yet they're blind to it as well. They're blind to it electively as they're instructed to by the industry that's orchestrated this whole ruse. That's the industry that's put their people in place, to afford them this control, Monsanto.

Well here's your news flash; sugar including carbs is addictive. That means that carbs are just an addictive food to eat as that of sugar. It's also deadly, deadlier than alcohol, deadlier than heroin, deadlier than cigarettes and drug addiction. Sugar addiction or ECC, (Excessive Carbohydrate Consumption) is responsible for more deaths than all world wars and terrorism combined. ECC is the deadliest addiction a person or society can have. Its toll on our society is massive, as it's responsible for over 2000 deaths every day in the US alone. That number jumps to over 50,000 worldwide (daily). The grief it creates is incalculable.

I can guarantee a manifestation of disease-causing AGEs to anyone who consumes a diet of grains. How much they consume will dictate how much glycation they get to deal with, but they will deal with it, guaranteed. The manner in which you cure the glycation will also cure the hunger. What it does to wipe out the hunger cycle (and it does it altogether), it also does to the glycation cycle. That is how you cure hunger.

That is also how you conquer and cure all modern diseases. You can do it in one fell swoop. This is exciting. To me, the cure for hunger is the same cure for all the modern diseases that are responsible for over 2000 deaths every day. If you cure one, you cure the other. That will go miles to cure the problem of hunger around the world. We need to stop supplying the world with our killing field grains. It's the hunger that proves the addictive nature of carbs. Once you break the addiction, you lose the hunger cycle and without a cycle to create your hunger, the hunger can't exist. Hunger is then cured. You just have to solve the problem of too many people going without nutritious food and being subjected to a diet of non-nutritious food, which includes the category of grains.

THANK YOU HUNGER!

It's the cycle of hunger that's responsible not only for growth, but also for all harm done in the name of growth or progress, as well as advancement, or security, or improvement. Those are all desires driven by the cycle of hunger. It's this cycle of hunger that drives these emotions. Deep down inside, you know this to be true. After you eat, when your blood sugars are at their highest, you are at one of your most relaxed attitudes of the day.

The only other times you feel this secure is right after you eat any meal or snack (unless you're consciously cheating on a diet and are dealing with guilt issues). This is the high side of the cycle, this is when you feel that everything is OK, "my stomach is full and I don't feel like I need anything except to sit here and relax for a minute. This is how you feel at the end of Thanksgiving Dinner, Christmas Dinner, New Years Day dinner, Easter Dinner, etc, etc, etc. This is also the end of every meal you eat, to some extent. This is the glucose hitting your bloodstream, waiting to give you fuel for energy. This is also the start of glycation and the hunger cycle.

It's the start of glycation because all that glucose you just put into your blood by eating your starchy grains, is now floating all through your blood after being broken down to glucose, starting with the saliva in your mouth. That means that before it hits your stomach, your blood glucose levels are reacting.

This is the start of the hunger cycle to which there is no end until you stop feeding it. When your blood glucose levels fall and your stomach starts to shrink just a little bit after the digestion of your meal, that triggers your stomach to release Ghrelin, your hunger hormone. That's the hormone that nobody on a carbohydrate diet can resist. That's because many of those on a carb diet must satisfy that Ghrelin hormone. Once they get hungry they feel the need to satisfy their hunger usually with some form of carbohydrate more than anything else. This is the low side of the cycle that drives people to abhorrent behavior because of their need.

This hunger and satiety cycle influences almost every other cycle our bodies go through. It's what's behind all the behavior, of those that are on a carbohydrate diet. This is the cycle that drives people into the use and abuse, of social media to slander, attack, and accuse without evidence, others they disagree with. As PBS's late **GWEN IFILL** said, "we have to guard against how we treat each other". We should remember it was cancer that took Gwen from us. If this cure had been publicized 10, 20, or 30 years ago, Gwen would still be here giving us her newscast.

This manner in how we treat each other is one of the reasons why I'm writing this book, about what this food source that Monsanto has given us to eat is doing to everyone who eats it. Up until I watched **FOOD, INC,** Monsanto only played a small part in my equation. I didn't realize they were behind this to the extent that they actually are. I now see that they are a much larger part of it than I suspected.

What their grains do with their glycating destruction starts with premature aging. It does that by driving fat production and the glycation factor that influences all modern disorders. That figures into everything glycation plays a factor in. Glycation is another name for inflammation. I know this. I've experienced the release of the addiction. The evidence in my books proves this. I know why we behave like the society that we do. It has to do with what we eat.

Nobody will believe me until they heed my advice and kick their own addiction. Only then, can they see the true light? I can guarantee the light you'll see is a light of freedom, true freedom. Freedom from the cycle of hunger that drives virtually every other cycle. If you can eliminate this cycle, you can eliminate everything this cycle creates and drives, starting with obesity and diabetes and moving on to glycation. That will go far to improve not only health, but mental attitudes, and hence better emotional outcomes and less strife.

That is true freedom, freedom from the cycle of hunger, freedom from the cycle of addiction. Freedom from the wild roller coaster ride of emotional swings. The freedom I experience is true freedom as this cycle does not affect anybody on a purely ketogenic diet. We're not subject to the hunger cycle that the carb diet requires. By the same token, we're not subject to the glycation cycle of destruction either. This cycle is also at the root of all violence and terrorism, as it's subject to the same hormonal changes that control your emotions, as explained above.

To control the glucose fluctuations, the easiest way is to control what feeds the cycle. That means to control the cycle you need to control the introduction of glucose into your body. Controlling the flow of sugars (carbs and fructose) is the only way you can control the blood glucose fluctuations.

As easy as this may sound, that may be furthest from the truth. Controlling the inflow of carbs into your body is as difficult as fighting any addiction, because that's exactly what you're doing, fighting an addiction. That's also why you must break the addiction, addictions kill prematurely and you can live without this addictive food. This brings me to the conclusion that a ketogenic diet is an optimal diet for a society to be following on, for the best health of that society. The ketogenic diet not only removes the hormonal control out of the equation, it removes hunger and glycation out of the equation. That makes it a truly win, win, win diet for everyone to follow.

The problem here is sticking to a ketogenic diet. We'll cover that here because it's not only important, it's vital to convert to the ketogenic diet to save yourself and our society as a whole. This is also how curing hunger can also cure terrorism by curing abhorrent behavior by removing your emotions from the hunger cycle. This removal of your emotions from the hunger cycle has multiple other benefits for your emotional behavior. It puts those emotions back in your control and not the control of the industry that promotes the masturbation of them. It also returns other emotional control you'd thought you'd lost years ago. The control you lost was a relinquishing of control to the industry that has addicted you. This isn't your fault. You've always eaten carbs and sugar. The fact that they were considered healthy at one time is an indication of their addictive nature. (If the body needs it, it must be healthy!) We now know, that science was skewed.

To be able to stick to a ketogenic diet means that you must break the addiction. Once it's broke, you'll know it and you'll know it firmly, distinctly. It's a feeling I still remember clearly, three years later. It's a feeling of freedom. It's a feeling of freedom from dependence on a substance that is as satisfying as it as dangerous.

That is what makes it so dangerous, the fact that is so satisfying, so satiating, so hormonal fluctuating. That also makes it emotionally fluctuating. That makes you prone to emotional outbursts and fits of terrorism, yourself. (Frightening people with the use of force is terrorism, by strict definition.) That makes any threat, terrorism, to some extent. Those who make the most threats (bullies) tend to be the most terroristic. If you control your emotions and not let what you eat control them, that gives you more control over your emotional reactions and the consequences of those emotional reactions. This is a small synopsis of the control that glucose has on your actions and reactions.

I, being on a ketogenic diet, do not experience this control of my emotions or actions or reactions due to glucose influence. I've learned how to live without that influence. I learned that three years, two weeks ago. It may have been the best day of my life. But I have to admit that sticking to a ketogenic diet is difficult to get into. It took me over two years to transform into the diet I've been on since I started writing my books.

One thing I know is that I could have never accomplished this without being on this diet. I've not only overcome severe chronic pain, but I've also overcome pre-diabetic conditions as well as high blood pressure, chronic constipation from the drugs that were prescribed, near obesity, and brain drain more than anything else. Being on my ketogenic diet has sharpened my brain to a point I wish it could have been when I was in school. Boy, would my life have been different? This is why I want to help you succeed at your attempt to convert, it's that important for our society if we're to end hunger and terrorism.

In order to do that, I recommend stopping buying everything that raises your blood glucose more than 50 pts on the glycemic index. This will help keep your blood glucose levels from reaching glycating or hunger cycling proportions. This is the starting point that I used when I started three years ago. I cut out bread first. That was the hardest because that included everything that flour is used in. To do otherwise is not giving up the bread. After the magic came from giving up the bread, I switched those calories to calories from higher fiber carbs like vegetables and fresh fruit. I was still reluctant to put dairy in my diet then, as I still have some Almond Milk in my fridge, I didn't realize it then because my knowledge hadn't grown to the point to where I decided to go completely ketogenic, so I was still putting more sugar in my body than what I am now, where I'm experiencing the improvements in my mental functions as well as my physical abilities. I'm actually healing my paralysis, little by little. My right side is actually getting more functional every day that I remain on this diet,

That is why I decided to convert to a completely keto diet after two years of simply a low carb diet. That may have got me to my weight goal, but it wasn't getting me my brain back. Quitting bread prompted me to quit all grains and starchy carbohydrates like potatoes and beans. That felt so great, I decided to go completely keto approximately one year ago. That's when I started my website and started writing all the information that I'm packing into three books. If anyone else were doing this I would think it phenomenal. But because it's myself doing this, I'm just driven to get this information out there where the public can see it. Killing my mother has become my driving force to get this known. My ability to accomplish this working in a state of paralysis, to me is what's phenomenal. For that, I have to thank Dr. Perlmutter. Thank you, Dr. Perlmutter, I couldn't have done this without your book or advice.

For those who want something to kill? I've got something for you to kill. Kill your hunger cycle. Kill it before it kills you first. Monsanto may have different ideas, though. Their profits depend on your hunger cycle. Their drug industry depends on your hunger cycle. Your hunger cycle drives you to eat more and more carbs to satisfy that hunger cycle. If you want to kill something worth killing, kill your hunger cycle and do it as quickly as you can. The following report from Wikipedia shows why;

- **The influence of funding on research and the management of conflicts of interests** as explained from The New England Journal of Medicine (Aug 19, 1993)

"*Conflict of interest" in the field of medical research has been defined as "a set of conditions in which professional judgment concerning a primary interest (such as a patients welfare or the validity of research) tends to be unduly influenced by a secondary interest (such as financial gain)."]*

In the early 1900s private companies such as the Carbolic Smoke Ball Company, Mrs. Winlow's Soothing Syrup among other snake medicine remedies were solicited around the world and were the cause of many deaths due to misinformation. Information was not readily available to consumers nor was it required of the pharmaceutical producers to inform their customers of the ingredients that they were consuming. Samuel Hopkins Adams was an investigator to uncover the wide corruption and falsehoods that existed within the American pharmaceutical industry. He is quoted saying: "Gullible America will spend this year some seventy-five millions of dollars in the purchase of patent medicines. In consideration of this sum, it will swallow huge quantities of alcohol, an appalling amount of opiates and narcotics, a wide assortment of varied drugs ranging from powerful and dangerous heart depressants to insidious liver stimulants; and far in excess of all other ingredients, undiluted fraud."

Regulation of industry-funded biomedical research has seen great changes since Samuel Hopkins Adams declaration. In 1906 Congress passed the Pure Food and Drugs Act of 1906. In 1912 Congress passed the Shirley Amendment to prohibit the wide dissemination of false information on pharmaceuticals. The Food and Drug Administration was formally created in 1930 under the McNairy Mapes Amendment to oversee the regulation of Food and Drugs in the United States. In 1962 the Kefauver-Harris Amendments to the Food, Drug, and Cosmetics Act made it so that before a drug was marketed in the United States the FDA must first approve that the drug was safe. The Kefauver-Harris amendments also mandated that more stringent clinical trials must be performed before a drug is brought to the market. The Kefauver-Harris amendments were met with opposition from industry due to the requirement of lengthier clinical trial periods that would lessen the period of time in which the investor is able to see a return on their money. In the pharmaceutical industry, patents are typically granted for a 20-year period of time, and most patent applications are submitted during the early stages of the product development. According to Ariel Katz on average after a patent application is submitted it takes an additional 8 years before the FDA approves a drug for marketing. As such this would leave a company with only 12 years to market the drug to see a return on their investments. After a sharp decline of new drugs entering the US market following the 1962 Kefauver-Harris amendments economist Sam Petlzman concluded that cost of loss of innovation was greater than the savings recognized by consumers no longer purchasing ineffective drugs. In 1984 the Hatch-Waxman Act or the Drug Price Competition and Patent Term Restoration Act of 1984 were passed by Congress. The Hatch-Waxman Act was passed with the idea that giving brand manufacturers the ability to extend their patent by an additional 5 years would create greater incentives for innovation and private sector funding for investment.

The relationship that exists with industry-funded biomedical research is that of which industry is the financier for academic institutions which in turn employ scientific investigators to conduct research. A fear that exists wherein a project is funded by industry is that firms might negate informing the public of negative effects to better promote their product. A list of studies shows that public fear of the conflicts of interest that exist when biomedical research is funded by industry can be considered valid after a 2003 publication of "Scope and Impact of Financial Conflicts of Interest in Biomedical Research" in The Journal of American Association of Medicine. This publication included 37 different studies that met specific criteria to determine whether or not an academic institution or scientific investigator funded by industry had engaged in behavior that could be deduced to be a conflict of interest in the field of biomedical research. Survey results from one study concluded that 43% of scientific investigators employed by a participating academic institution had received research-related gifts and discretionary funds from industry sponsors. Another participating institution surveyed showed that 7.6% of investigators were financially tied to research sponsors, including paid speaking engagements (34%), consulting arrangements (33%), advisory board positions (32%) and equity (14%). A 1994 study concluded that 58% out of 210 life science companies indicated that investigators were required to withhold information pertaining to their research as to extend the life of the interested companies' patents. Rules and regulations regarding conflict of interest disclosures are being studied by experts in the biomedical research field to eliminate conflicts of interest that could possibly affect the outcomes of biomedical research.

This is pretty much the definition of what Monsanto has accomplished in the last 40-50 years and they seem to be doing their level best to increase their power and influence. It's their food that glycates your blood. It's their food that addicts you to eat more and more of their food. It's their food that creates the hunger cycle that drives your behavior. It's this company that is forcing farmers to purchase their seed to grow the crops to put on your table to eat. That means that it's this company that is responsible for over 45,000 deaths every day, across the world from ECC, Excessive Carbohydrate Consumption. ECC is the deadliest addiction mankind has ever been exposed to. Monsanto, who's infiltrated their execs into the offices of the USDA and the FDA and the departments that control all the agencies and offices within them, controls all. From planting to harvesting to processing to treating, Monsanto has their hands in everything. Can you trust a corporation that's dedicated to owning your hunger? If they own your hunger, they own you.

This has given them unprecedented control over what you eat. That has given them full control over the diseases and disorders, all who eat their food will acquire. That is something I can virtually guarantee. Why? It lies in the science of a glucose diet, the deadliest diet man can eat. Thank you, Monsanto, but I disrespectfully decline your offer to buy your drugs and live life as you see fit.

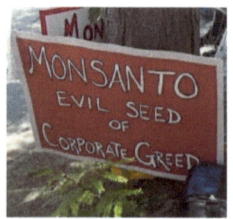

I CHOOSE THE WAY FORWARD

PART III

A NEW TOMORROW

CHAPTER 9

FASTING AND THE KETOGENIC DIET

As far back as 500BC, physicians have used fasting as a means to find the way back to health by a simple and inexpensive manner in which one could actually heal themselves from virtually any of the modern diseases that have plagued man since the dawn of civilization. For me, it's easy to see the correlation of the emergence of modern diseases with the gradual increase of consumption of einkorn wheat, the precursor to our modern strains of wheat. From Emmer (one of the first domesticated strains) and Durum Semolina which is little higher in gluten (yet it's still considered a weak wheat as the wheat doesn't rise as well as it holds the dough together to hold the pasta shape.) Winter Red, spelt and other bread wheat or common wheat that are higher in gluten have been used for bread for thousands of years because they rise better.

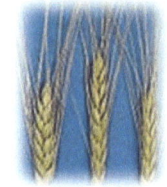

Today's forms of highly modified wheat act nothing like the strains from thousands of years ago as today's *highly domesticated strains of wheat cannot survive in the wild.* That's according to Wikipedia and that's due to their inability to disperse their seeds. Monsanto has made certain of that through their genetic modifying to create ender seeds that won't get pollinated so a farmer has no seed for next year's crop forcing them to buy GMO seed from Monsanto. (GMO by itself is not dangerous. It's what the modifying allows the farmer to do that makes it dangerous and that's to spray it with Roundup. Their seed is genetically modified to handle applications of the glyphosate herbicide.) This is the wheat that Monsanto is forcing their farmers to grow for your cereal, bread, and snacks. The same glyphosate exists in the cornfields as well, contaminating every corn chip that you eat. (When was the last time you ate Mexican food?)

But we're talking about wheat right now which was originally cultivated in the Fertile Crescent 10,000 years ago, approximately the same time that modern disease started showing up in the bones of the remains of the people. This is a clear indication of the glycation that wheat was responsible for, even then, even as slow as the einkorn wheat is to digest (which slows the progression of glycation). The glycation existed then as it does now, only it took it much longer to manifest. Today, it manifests itself immediately (as soon as it touches your tongue) and this is due to the fast dissolving gluten flour that's used for bread and pastries as well as pasta and cereal. It glycates more now as the grain has changed immensely in the last 10,000 years. As this food increased in prevalence in our diet, the rates of disease increased, as it's these grains that have always generated disease. They generate it so slowly that it's never noticed until it's too late or you stop eating it. This is the value of fasting and why fasting is so important to the health of anyone on this type of carbohydrate diet.

This is why fasting has always cured disease. 98% of all disease is a direct result of our diet. With that being said, it's easy to see why removing everything damaging from our diet is going to heal the damage caused by keeping those foods in the diet. Fasting produces such good results it's been the subject of over 20,000 studies on PMC in the NLM at the NIH. (PMC has reported from across the world. PubMed has 590 reports from studies done in the US alone.) It's that important, yet what has your doctor shared with you about this life-saving course of intervention? Your doctor comes into your appointed meeting with his/her prescription tablet in hand ready to prescribe pharmaceuticals. Their whole intent is to prescribe drugs for your ailments, which are more than likely caused by the ingestion of grain foods. Prescribing drugs is the way they're trained to treat patients, not with recommendations for diet. (Monsanto wouldn't allow that to take place as they have far more control over your life than what you could ever believe.)

That's exactly why fasting is so healthy. It removes the worst of the toxins in our bodies that are built up from the diets of bread, wheat, and grain-based products, and doesn't put more toxins back in with the prescribed drugs. Those grain products also happen to be the most addictive, which is what makes them the hardest to give up. The addictive nature of sugar, at its worst, is displayed in this manner (when it drives pharmaceuticals). When one fasts, they give up the sugars that are doing all the glycating and it's this glycation that is at the root of all disease and this is why going without food is so healthy.

It also sets your body up for future health by resetting the hormonal structure in your body. This is mostly the result of your hormones transitioning to a starvation mode of survival, where the Ghrelin your stomach releases, sends this growth hormone throughout your body allowing it to do its magic in repairing damage and extending cell life where cell death took place before. (This is directly due to the carbohydrate influence in the diet, creating glycation.) It's the elimination of glycation that initially brings back a resemblance of health but that's not what brings future health. It's the breaking of an addiction. This addiction is built into our society so much, It starts in our prenatal body and continues through the first year of life and then on. (This is due to the prevalence of sugar and high fructose corn syrup in baby foods, formula, and infant medicines.) The prenatal effect starts with mama's diet before you're born, if your mother ate carbs, you got them before you were born. But that only explains why you're dependent. It doesn't explain how to break the dependence. That's with fasting and the keto diet, or ketogenic diet (the diet our ancestors were on, ever since our existence). The keto diet involves fasting as part of the diet, making it much easier to maintain. (There's no hunger.) Fasting does that by sending your body into ketosis.

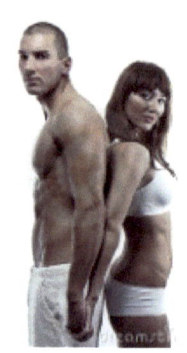

According to Wikipedia; in the early 20th century around 1911; Bernarr Macfadden, an American exponent of physical culture, popularized the use of fasting to restore health. His disciple, the osteopathic physician Hugh Conklin, of Battle Creek, Michigan, began to treat his epilepsy patients by recommending fasting. Conklin conjectured that epileptic seizures were caused when a toxin, secreted from the Peyer's patches in the intestines, was discharged into the bloodstream. Conklin's fasting therapy was adopted by neurologists in mainstream practice. In 1916, a Dr. McMurray wrote to the New York Medical Journal claiming to have successfully treated epilepsy patients with a fast, followed by a starch-and sugar-free diet, since 1912. In 1921, prominent endocrinologist H. Rawle Geyelin reported his experiences to the American Medical Association convention. He had seen Conklin's success first-hand and had attempted to reproduce the results in 36 of his own patients. He achieved similar results despite only having studied the patients for a short time. He reported that three water-soluble compounds, β-

hydroxybutyrate, acetoacetate and acetone (known collectively as ketone bodies), were produced by the liver in otherwise healthy people when they were starved or if they consumed a very low-carbohydrate, high-fat diet.

With fasting being able to eliminate so many disorders, a path was sought to bring this form of healing to the mainstream by creating a diet to encourage fasting. Thus the ketogenic diet was born in 1921 through the efforts of Russel Wilder. According to Wikipedia, Russel Wilder, at the Mayo Clinic, built on this research and coined the term ketogenic diet to describe a diet that produced a high level of ketone bodies in the blood (ketonemia) through an excess of fat and lack of carbohydrate.

Fasting is the quickest manner in which to allow your body to go into ketosis, yet it may not be the easiest. Although on second thought, being the quickest way may make it the easiest. I went through two weeks of withdrawal because I couldn't give up all the foods I loved to eat all at once, to allow my body to go into ketosis in a few days. I could have avoided 10 days of want by fasting and only want something to eat for a few days, as what happens when you fast for a minimum of 3 days. A longer fast is more beneficial but the three days allows your body to respond by going into ketosis which is a fat burning mode. It's this fat burning mode that forces your body to make its own glucose, which is a much cleaner glucose than you get from the sugar you eat, as it's a clean glucose made from your own glycogen or fat storage. Getting into ketosis quicker could allow you to start your fat burning diet, but continuing some carbs will only make the withdrawal more difficult as it may drop your body back out of ketosis. This was my problem and why my transition took so long. (Thankfully, they'll be no next time.)

Ketosis refers to acids in the body that are derived and used while in a state of low glucose in the blood. Because my body has been in a state of ketosis for the last 3 years, I feel qualified to speak about this lifestyle. I call it a lifestyle because it really is. It's a lifestyle completely different from the lifestyle of a carboholic. Carboholics require food every other hour or so, it's the law of glucose consumption, appetite follows glucose levels in the blood. It's that simple, blood sugar levels rise and satiety sets in, releasing hormones controlling feel-good emotions influencing behavior. But, that usually happens when the blood sugars fall again after a couple hours releasing hormones of hunger, need and want. These hormones are completely different than the satiety hormones and have a much different effect on the body, sometimes unrecognizable behavioral effects.

This is where carboholics do not have the advantage that ketonemiacs have. Ketonemiacs (those who have allowed their bodies to go into a state of ketosis) aren't controlled by their hormones, so they don't have to follow any hunger cycle. They're in full control of their hormones. This also means that they're in more control of their emotions because of that. I know that it doesn't sound like it's that big of a deal, but it's more important than you could ever imagine. First, let's look at the state of ketosis, as explained in Wikipedia;

"**Ketosis** is a metabolic state in which most of the body's energy supply comes from **ketone bodies** in the blood, in contrast to a state of **glycolysis** in which **blood glucose** provides most of the energy. Ketosis is similar to a condition called **KETOACIDOSIS**, in that both cause a side effect known to laypeople as **acetone breath**."

"Longer-term ketosis may result from **fasting** or staying on a low-carbohydrate diet, and deliberately induced ketosis serves as a medical intervention for various conditions, such as intractable epilepsy, and the various types of diabetes. In glycolysis, higher levels of insulin promote storage of body fat and block the release of fat from adipose tissues, while in ketosis, fat reserves are readily released and consumed. For this reason, ketosis is sometimes referred to as the body's "fat burning" mode."

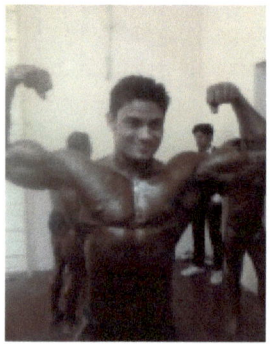

Even bodybuilders have recognized ketonemia or ketosis as being the most beneficial state to keep their body in as it's in this state where they produce more growth hormones because of the amount of Ghrelin their stomachs release to enable them to grow their muscles bigger without the carbs.

The state of ketosis is often confused with a state of ketoacidosis, which has nothing to do with being in a state of nutritional ketosis. Ketoacidosis is a state of extreme ketosis that can only happen to type 1 diabetics because their pancreas is incapable of secreting enough insulin to handle the amount of glucose in their system. Because of this the liver of type 1 diabetics secretes more ketones than what the body needs to operate. What if the glucose never made it into the system?

Although I appreciate ketosis as being a "fat burning mode", it's the other benefits that I appreciate more. Benefits like less pain, no headaches, no stomachaches, far more energy than what I've ever had, ability to get more work done, as I don't have to stop all the time to eat and although I do eat at my desk, I'm usually at my desk 16-18 hours out of the day, except on therapy days. I like to take 3 hours, 3 days a week for therapy. My therapy is exercise. My brain needs it, but my body benefits. Again Wikipedia says on the subject of ketosis;

*"Ketosis is deliberately induced by use of a **ketogenic diet** as a medical intervention in cases of intractable **epilepsy**. Other uses of **low-carbohydrate diets** remain controversial. Induced ketosis or low-carbohydrate diet terms have very wide interpretation. Therefore, Stephen S. Phinney and Jeff S. Volek coined the term "nutritional ketosis" to avoid the confusion.*

*"Ketoacidosis is a metabolic state associated with high concentrations of **ketone bodies**, formed by the breakdown of fatty acids and the **deamination** of **amino acids**. Ketoacidosis is most common in untreated **type 1 diabetes mellitus** when the liver breaks down **fat** and proteins in response to a perceived need for a **respiratory substrate**. Prolonged alcoholism may lead to alcoholic ketoacidosis. "*

*"In **diabetic ketoacidosis**, a high concentration of ketone bodies is usually accompanied by **insulin** deficiency, **hyperglycemia**, and **dehydration**. Particularly in type 1 diabetics the lack of insulin in the bloodstream prevents **glucose** absorption, thereby inhibiting the production of **oxaloacetate** (a crucial precursor to the β-oxidation of fatty acids) through reduced levels of **pyruvate** (a byproduct of **glycolysis**), and can cause unchecked ketone body production (through fatty acid metabolism) potentially leading to dangerous glucose and ketone levels in the blood. Hyperglycemia results in glucose overloading the **kidneys** and **spilling into the urine** (transport maximum for glucose is exceeded). Dehydration results following the osmotic movement of water into **urine**. (Osmotic diuresis), exacerbates the **acidosis**."*

"I bring this up to make the point that nutritional ketosis is not ketoacidosis. It's far from it. According to Wikipedia again, *"Normal **serum reference ranges** for ketone bodies are 0.5–3.0 mg/dL, equivalent to 0.05–0.29 mmol/L.[23]"* In ketosis, the levels range from 3 – 6 mg/dL. Ketoacidosis requires a level of 15 – 25 mg/dL, more the three times needed for ketosis, making it virtually impossible for anyone to into ketoacidosis if you're not a type 1 diabetic. Type 1 diabetics are required to make sure their bodies don't produce many ketones because of the risk of ketoacidosis".

According to **PMC's report** on Calorie Restriction (CR) or fasting, submitted; July 2010; *Nevertheless, ongoing research continues to draw a more complete picture of CR at the molecular level, which may ultimately allow for the development of therapeutics that might be able to confer at least some of the health benefits of this dietary regimen.*

Ketosis, being based on fasting, makes it the optimal diet for anybody to be on. Remaining in a state of ketosis has allowed my body to regain that which was lost 31 years ago in the car accident that left me severely disabled because of a severe closed head injury, (it was the two strokes that were the most devastating.)

It's become evident to me since I've been carb free and in a state of ketonemia or ketosis, how much our society is addicted to this drug, sugar, that does little more than to lead those who eat it to further drug use. Our food industrial complex sees to that by their advertising. I'm convinced it's because they're associated with the pharmaceutical industry. They used to be merged into one corporation that controlled the seed supply for the farmers as well as the chemicals to spray on the crops and the pharmaceuticals that treated to pain and discomfort brought on by the products made by the grains grown by those crops, made with the seed Monsanto sold to the farmer, and sprayed multiple times with glyphosate herbicide. (Yeah that was a mouthful, yet it wasn't the worst of it.) Two weeks before harvest, the crop gets desiccated to ensure higher yield in their harvest. This may be great for the farmer and Monsanto, but it ensures more than that. It ensures that it gets into your diet and into your body.

The unfortunate result of this love affair with those snack and comfort foods is what this diet brings, at its cost of this pleasure. The price to be paid is in the discomfort that this food brings to all those who eat it, regardless of how much they eat. The food industry (Monsanto in particular) has a fortune invested in maintaining your appetite for this deadly food. They've built an industry just to treat diabetes, with all the glucose meters and pumps out there, just so addicts can get their next fix. The trouble this industry goes to just to keep their addicts happy and addicted is unsurpassed in any field.

I know now what I didn't 4 years ago when I was an addict. The amount an addict consumes at each sitting dictates how much damage it's going to do, but it's going to do damage. There is no way to avoid it. That's the way our digestion and metabolism works. That's why this addiction is by far, the worst addiction our society has to deal with. This addiction leads to every other addiction that we're actively fighting, including alcoholism, heroin and tobacco and even gambling. Yes, even gambling is driven by the glucose addiction, as gambling is driven by the hunger cycle which is one of the biggest underlying influences of a carbohydrate diet. Hunger in this diet drives absolutely everything, even breathing, and because of that, eventually drugs.

This is a cycle that I don't need. As a matter of fact, it's the last thing I need. (You don't need it either.)The biggest reason I refuse to take any of these drugs anymore is that all of them carry side effects, some major, some minor. Whether the side effects are major or minor, I don't want to experience any of them, anymore. I've had my fill of side effects, especially the ones that make my health worse, which is where most of these side effects should be classified. That only invites more treatment, which in turn invites more of my money into the pockets of the pharmaceutical industry. This is a cycle that I can't afford to be part of anymore.

After living for twenty years needing to take massive amounts of opioids for my chronic severe pain, diuretics for my high blood pressure, anti-depressants for the pain, and living with the side effects of not only the opioids, but every other drug they had me on, all twelve of them, I got fed up with it. I wasn't going to take it anymore as I just couldn't afford it. And I was only up to twelve medications. I have a friend who's on this diet, who's lowered his needs to thirteen daily medications from twenty-three. How many meds do you take every day? How many would you like to do without, if your health would allow? This is where fasting needs to replace ~~doping~~ dosing. A change in diet will go much further than any drug and the cure lasts longer than any treatment.

I prefer to live by the theory that if the meds aren't needed in the first place, my health is going to be that much better. That is why I removed everything from my diet that I could that's responsible for these horrendous diseases, which require the need for these medications. By fasting, one can reach this healing state much quicker than I did, just by cutting out my bread. Where it took me two weeks to get into full ketosis, by fasting I could have jump-started the state by starving my body, then go on from there with my ketogenic diet to keep my body in this healing state.

Case in point about fasting, in this report, dated April 22, 2010, on the effects of a ketogenic diet on glioblastoma multiforme;

Abstract

Background

Management of glioblastoma multiforme (GBM) has been difficult using standard therapy (radiation with temozolomide chemotherapy). The ketogenic diet is used commonly to treat refractory epilepsy in children and, when administered in restricted amounts, can also target energy metabolism in brain tumors. We report the case of a 65-year-old woman who presented with progressive memory loss, chronic headaches, nausea, and a right hemisphere multi-centric tumor seen with magnetic resonance imaging (MRI). Following incomplete surgical resection, the patient was diagnosed with glioblastoma multiforme expressing hypermethylation of the MGMT gene promoter.

Results

After two months treatment, the patient's body weight was reduced by about 20% and no discernable brain tumor tissue was detected using either FDG-PET or MRI imaging. Biomarker changes showed reduced levels of blood glucose and elevated levels of urinary ketones. MRI evidence of tumor recurrence was found 10 weeks after suspension of strict diet therapy.

Conclusion

This is the first report of confirmed GBM treated with standard therapy together with a restricted ketogenic diet. As rapid regression of GBM is rare in older patients following incomplete surgical resection and standard therapy alone, the response observed in this case could result in part from the action of the calorie restricted ketogenic diet. Further studies are needed to evaluate the efficacy of restricted ketogenic diets, administered alone or together with standard treatment, as a therapy for GBM and possibly other malignant brain tumors.

The question I ask the industry here is, why is this information known by so few people? This report was dated April 2010. That's over 7 years ago and I've not heard anything about this until I found it in my research. How many people know to research this? How many that have cancer know? How many have died since then?

Actually, more and more people are beginning to recognize the value of the ketogenic diet. The time may be for you to find out for yourself. If you're fighting cancer, I highly recommend it. What's got to lose? Your addiction, your pain, your bad health?

This is where the advantage of fasting reveals it's butterfly from the cocoon of fasting, it not only starts the healing from the beginning by putting your body in a starvation mode, it allows you to stay in that mode for the rest of your life. That one little option in itself is what's going to extend your life beyond 100 years. I can see where ultimately man will be able to extend its lifespan to over 150 years old. !00 years from now, when all mankind is on a ketogenic or paleo diet again, I can see the oldest people in the world living into their 180's, doubling today's extended lifespan.

This can be easily obtained simply by allowing our bodies to heal themselves and not keep depending on drugs for the perception of healing, which ultimately brings nothing but more drug use, which ultimately is what ruins the liver and kidneys leading to all the cancers and disorders of the hepatic and renal systems. This drug dependence is driven by another dependence that we've all been born into.

I hope that you're beginning to see how our drug addictions are driven by one thread that drives all modern diseases along with it. That one thread is what ties 100% of all cancers, 98% of all heart diseases, and 99.9 % of all dementia, all arthritis, all headaches, and almost all stomach aches together is one substance that can be removed from the diet without any severe side effects.

I shouldn't need to tell you what that substance is by now. You should know. You eat it every day and you live with the effects of its addiction every day. Pain always comes with addiction. (That's what makes breaking the addiction so rewarding, limiting the pain cycle. Oh, what sweet bliss! Ending a cycle well worth ending.) The idea then is to limit to minuscule amounts, the foods that make up these addictive substances. You should know by now what these foods are, you eat them every morning, either in your coffee as creamer, in the toast you have, or the cereal you consume. You have it every lunch with your sandwich or burrito and with every dinner with your rolls.

I have known several families that would just put a plate of bread on the table every evening. This is the display of addiction, a full out need to satisfy the taste buds by dumping more and more sugar in the body, usually in the form of the starchy carbs of bread. I've also noticed that in those houses that served bread there was always beer cans in the garbage indicating another addiction.

If you remove this one addiction from our society, you remove all addictions, as this addiction to sugar and carbs is the foundation of all other addictions as they are all based on a hunger cycle which is the result of an addiction to sugar. Do you think, that might make it the root of all evil? Maybe we should ask John Barleycorn.

I hope that you can see now that it's this addiction to sugar and carbs that are enriching the pharmaceutical industry, and that both industries are driven by the same people who have and keep a major influence in the offices of the agencies that are supposed to regulate this industry, the FDA, the USDA, the CDC and the EPA. With that kind of influence, there's only one way to fight it and that's to not buy into it.

To not buy into it does require a diet of grain abstinence, though. That requires breaking the addiction and moving to as much of a ketogenic diet, as possible. The easiest manner to do this is to do a strict three day, water only fast. The longer you can do it the better, but it must be at least 3 days with absolutely no food. That's why it's important to check with your doctor first.

It's the consumption of the grain industry's products that are driving the pharmaceutical industry's profits today and will drive it tomorrow, next year, and for the next 500 and beyond. If we don't put an end to this now, our society is doomed to suffer the consequences of a carbohydrate addiction that no one is responsible for, for the rest of time.

The greed of the grain industry combined with the ambition of the pharmaceutical industry has made us all carboholic slaves to the desires of these industries. It's these industries that are rewarding from the most, from this arrangement. For me, it's scary, how much power we've given these industries, simply because we listen to their advertising. We've also let them take over the regulating agency that's supposed to control this industry. Because our health depends on it, we can't allow Monsanto to dictate how there are going to poison our food, so they can bolster the profits of the pharmaceutical industry. Not knowing what you put in your body can cost you your life. It is costing you your life if you eat carbs. Those who listen to the advertising and are influenced by it, fall prey to that influence and become their slaves for life or until they quit consuming the grains. There's very little difference than that of alcoholism except that it's pretty much forced upon us, in our baby food. Mamas, feed your babies on your own milk if you want them to be healthy (and make sure there's no extra lactose in it from the glucose that you eat in your carbs).

I know what you're thinking right now, what are all the foods involved in this addiction? The list is enormous and that's why this is such a dangerous addiction. This industry has virtually forced us to celebrate this addiction. It involves every one of our holidays, with the holiday season being the worst. Every celebration involves some form of sugar. From the Sugar Bowl to the Tostido's Fiesta Bowl, our celebration is never-ending. Just after the "holiday season" comes Valentine's Day barely a month later. Then, comes Easter and spring break. Are you beginning to understand why this addiction is our worst? With all the celebrating we need to keep this addiction, how do you change tradition without changing the world? The quickest way that I know is to organize an international health weekend, for 3 days, where everyone goes keto to heal their diseases and give their bodies a chance to go into ketosis, the ever healing state of metabolism.

The best advantage of this diet is the amount of control it gives you over your own emotions. You may think that you control your emotions right now, but I can tell you with full confidence, if you're on a carb diet, you have no control over your emotions. They're completely controlled by what you eat because what you eat controls your hunger cycle and it's your hunger cycle that drives every other cycle your body goes through.

Since your hunger cycle is controlled by your hormones (mostly leptin and Ghrelin), it's these hormones that are controlling your emotions. You know this every time you crave that bagel or biscotti. Once you bite into it, your saliva starts digesting that instantly gratifying food to give you that *aww* feeling, that instantly hits your brain, even before you can swallow it. This is your first sign of addiction and dependence that only gives you the perception that you have control of your own emotions. It's this cycle that is in full control of your emotions. As much as you try to control them, too often they have a tendency to slip out of your control and back into theirs.

Anyone who can't control their emotions entirely by themselves is a slave to their own hormones. This makes every carboholic a slave to their emotions and therefore a slave to these industries. This displays the dependence of the hunger cycle and the carb diet that drives that hunger cycle. You may not classify these as emotions, but I submit that they actually are. Satiety is defined as the state of being satisfied. If that is not an emotion, as it expresses feelings of calmness and security, I don't know what is. Hunger, on the other hand, is defined as a strong desire. Is not that an emotion? These emotions are controlled by both leptin and ghrelin, which ultimately are controlled by the grain industry, more than anything else. This is the ruse I refuse to take part in. I can't afford this trap anymore. The only way out for our society is to break the hold of this industry, to let them know that we're not going to stand for this kind of abuse. To go ketogenic in your diet is the best way you can get yourself to everlasting health.

With emotions being controlled by our hormonal balance like this, it's easy to see how carbs could influence that balance. For this to not have an effect on our behavior is beyond comprehension. It has to. When you combine the drive of an addiction (which is what we're talking about) with the advertisements promoting that addiction, how can it not have an effect on our health and ultimately our society? That is why I make the statement that this cycle has to change. If it doesn't cease, our health as a society will never get better. There's never been a better time for a cure, and that cure is a ketogenic diet, not only for each and everybody to be as healthy as possible, but also to regain the health of our whole society. Can you imagine a world where everyone not only controls their own emotions but they're in control of their emotions? (That includes reactions.)

Let's go back to addiction, though, for you may still not consider this an addiction. I understand few caught in an addiction can recognize that addiction when they're feeding it because the addiction has ways of hiding itself. You can ask anyone who has to have at least one beer a day. They're not addicted to their beer, as far as they're concerned, yet they have to have it. And often they don't even drink more than just one. But they still have to have that one. That is what makes it an addiction.

The body can and does live much better without beer, so it's not a substance the body requires to survive. Yet the beer drinker needs that daily beer to satisfy their addiction. To go without, many times creates more problems because of the work your hormones are doing on your emotions and worse yet your actions, by controlling how receptors work in your brain. That makes it a natural thing that you need to do, and not an addiction, to appease that desire to drink the beer. This is how addiction works and it happens to carboholics too. I know I am a carboholic. The desire for sweets is still with me. It's the last refuge of my addiction. It's something that I get to fight for the rest of my life.

The fact of the matter is, if you were fed baby food, you've been fed sugar, simply to get you to swallow it. This addicted you to glucose immediately. Actually, you've been sold the idea that sugar and carbs were healthy foods to eat. The fault was found with every other type of nutrition except grains, until recent history. For more than 60 years, we've been told to eat grains. Thirty years ago, they said whole grains are healthy. They still say "whole grains are healthy", yet according to all the studies I've seen out of the hundreds I've looked at, nothing about this food is safe to ingest, leaving me to wonder, why do they still recommend it? Then I look at who controls the FDA, the USDA and what interest they have in their industrial farming, and it becomes pretty clear whose influence this is, controlling what we eat.

This simple little act of feeding your baby formula laced with sugars to get you to eat it has addicted you to a lifetime of dependence. It addicted me. Even though I broke the addiction, I'm still affected by what control it did have over me. That's exactly why I'm pleading with you, don't let it control you. I can virtually guarantee that you won't like the end results. Whether they come sooner or later, they always come. (They're as dependable as the tide.)

When I think about this, my first response is to get angry, for I never asked for this, nor could I ever wish it upon anyone else. Yet, there is an industry that is committed to not only continuing this cycle, they're goal is to increase its scope and they're doing it on an exponential basis. You can see this in all the advertising. It's affecting you. You can see that in the rates of cancer deaths, CVD deaths, dementia deaths, etc, etc.

This is your grain industry pushing this celebration of this addiction and you're buying into it every time you feed your carb diet, by buying all your snacks, pasta, cereal, soft drinks, and beer, just for starters. I'd go on with the rest but space limits that list in this book. You can find it in both my first and second books, *It's Time for a Cure* and *Time for the Ultimate Cure*. Your best guide is to use the glycemic index as your guide for what foods that are safe to eat or not. It's the general consensus that you should keep your foods lower than 50 on the glycemic index.

My contention is to keep carbs out of your diet completely and let your body make its own glucose. The reason you want to keep your blood glucose low is to avoid the hunger cycle. The hunger cycle is emotionally the worst manifestation of a carb diet. As it controls your emotions, it controls your actions and reactions. This is an undeniable truth. You know it as well as I do. You feel it every time you taste that divine taste when you bite into it, MMM how good it is.

This is where you need to ask yourself, what is it you crave most? If what you crave has any carbohydrate in it, then that's your first indication that you're addicted. What kind of carb you crave, quite often tells how bad your addiction is. One wouldn't think that a hamburger could be a sign of addiction, when actually when you think about the taste you crave, it's a combination of everything including the bun, which happens to be the addictive ingredient in the hamburger. Everything else in the hamburger is healthy. It's just the gluten in the bun that's so addictive. I wouldn't doubt that they use extra high gluten bread dough for the buns used for these sandwiches, as it's more addictive, due to the high gluten content. I know they use high gluten bread dough for making pizza dough because it needs to rise, and the more the gluten the better it rises. That makes it taste better, but it also makes it more addictive. That's why when you're at one of these restaurants, most everyone there is overweight. They're there because they crave that high gluten bread dough. You get it in both pizzas and fast food hamburgers. This is how they make you repeat customers.

If you think my assessment is wrong, just try eating your favorite hamburger between two slices of lettuce. The taste is completely different. Most fast food restaurants offer low carb sandwiches but few order them. The only ones that I know of who order them are those who suffer from celiac disease and I believe that all of us suffer somewhat from celiac disease. I think that there are only a very few that can get through life without showing or suffering the effects of a carb diet....especially an excessive carb diet as in the case with most people worldwide today.

The reason you crave the taste of a hamburger is that of the high gluten bread dough the buns are made from because it's that bun that raises your blood glucose as soon as it hits your tongue. Therein lies the addictive nature of glucose, the constant tug on your hunger cycle. It's caused by the foods you eat if you're on a carb diet. When you stop to think about it, you know it, as well as I.

You just need to do something about it, as I did, three years ago, and then again one year ago when I went complete keto. It took me three years to go completely keto. You can do it in one month if you've got the guts to do a thirty day fast. I didn't and I may have suffered because of it. I guess I was still persuaded to eat the carbs even after I gave up the bread. If I had to do it over again, I'd fast, to go keto. The adjustment is a lot quicker.

What do you think they're advertising when they show you those commercials for pizza and their soft drinks, fruit drinks, cereals, bread, pasta, pastries, candy, etc, etc? They selling you that mmm feeling of dependence and addiction. It's that feeling you get as soon as your favorite food hits your tongue and makes you go "ooh, I needed that". That's the same feeling a junkie feels when he gets his latest fix.

That is precisely why this food can't sustain us in space and that's why the keto diet is so important. For our species to travel into space, we'll have to do away with the hunger cycle altogether.

SPACE TRAVEL WILL REQUIRE A KETOGENIC DIET RATHER THAN A CARBOHYDRATE DIET.

To me, this is simple, yet almost impossible to see when you're stuck in the addiction that's responsible for the reason. Again, it's a matter of how the food is digested. Carbs ultimately create glycation. Fats and proteins don't. It's that simple. That and the fact that this food creates a hunger cycle that can't be controlled without ending their consumption. One needs to compare the value of the food, in respects to the number of calories per gram of nutrition. Carbs have 4 calories whereas fat has 9, per gram of nutrition. This is important to remember as it's the calories that are important to have.

Your body requires calories to survive, so it's important to know where you're getting your calories from? Are you getting more calories from less food or do you need to eat more food to get an adequate amount of calories? Carb diets require more food per calorie, plus they're the highest calorie count of any diet. Because carbs incite hunger, they require massive amounts of calories to sustain, due to leptin resistance. This hunger cycle is a cycle that should be avoided at all costs, as it's the cycle that's at the root of all evil cycles as well. This cycle will prove to be an unsustainable cycle in space, as it does little more than to create disease in the body. Instead of using your hormones to heal the body, you're using your hormones to damage the body.

This is because the body is producing insulin and using it to turn the glucose into fat. While creating insulin, the body has little reason to create glucagon, the opposite of insulin. It's the glucagon that helps create your growth hormones. The glucagon is generated during times of hunger and fasting. Ghrelin influences how much glucagon your body makes by how much insulin you use. This is the nature of leptin resistance and explains why it's important to make yourself ghrelin resistant.

That makes the type of food you eat important, very import. Is the food you eat the most "high octane" or is it low octane "dirty fuel"? Is it clean burning fat or is it dirty burning fat? If it's fat from carbs, it's going to be dirty at best. That's if you're lucky enough for it not to be polluted with glyphosate. But then, by the time we're ready to travel that far into the stars, hopefully, we'll be past the glucose ruse and the glyphosate scourge that's the evil part of it.

If Love wins out and we're able to travel to the stars with everybody on a ketogenic diet, our world will truly be a different one then. It'll no longer be a world that's a slave to the hunger cycle and all the evil that can bring. Instead, it will be a world that can see past fear and anger. It'll be a world free of suspicion and fear. I will be an all-inclusive world, with one exception, the corporate evil that exists today because of the hunger cycle will be replaced by cycles of benevolence and charity, with more intent to help than profit. Corporations in the future will break free of the hunger cycle of profit and loss and learn that true profit can only be long-term in which the benefits are available for all mankind and not just a few stockholders. (You have to break free from the addiction to see this.)

But to explain more succinctly why we can't eat carbs in space;

1. We'd have to grow them. Where are we going to get the water to grow them? I know there are some polar ice caps on Mars, but I don't think that's going to be enough for 100's of years until we get the technology to transport the water to where we can use it to harvest crops. Those crops though, are going to inflict the same harm that they've been inflicting for 10,000 years, and that's through the glycation they create. That's going to require medication to fight

the pain created by the glycation. That is a senseless proposition.
2. The hunger cycle requires feeding every 3-4 hours or at least 3 times a day, not including snacks.
3. Without a hunger cycle, there are no snacks. There's only one meal per day (if you want that one).
4. There's much less waste from the digestion process. lessening the need for sanitation supplies. This is because there's only one meal, and it's a small one, just a little protein, and a little fat.
5. We'd have to take medication for all the problems carbs do to the body. That digestion can't be changed in less than a couple thousand years, our DNA won't let it. We'll be required to address everything in space that we address right here on earth, in regards to what sugar does to the body. That influence must be removed, from any diet of a space traveler.
6. A ketogenic diet gives the body a repairing diet that will be much more advantageous where medical treatment will be limited, at best. The sensible diet to be on is one that doesn't generate any glycation or hunger, yet generates growth hormones, instead. A diet that promotes brain growth instead of brain disease will go a lot further for our species' travels in space. This is why I can only recommend our species as a whole to go on a ketogenic diet.
7. A diet of carbs will come with a diet with glyphosate in it. Glyphosate is toxic. It's carcinogenic, atherosclerotic and extremely inflammatory. This is unsustainable off of this planet, without the resources that will be needed to treat all the pain that will be created by this glyphosated, carbohydrate diet.
8. Carbohydrates will not be available without the glyphosate sprayed on them, for at least 50 if not 100 years from now. The earth may not heal from the glyphosate contamination for 500 years, if then.
9. The carb diet creates fear cycles as a result of the hunger cycle. Combine that with the brain disease the carbs create and that's a recipe for disaster. That's the maker of every phobia and mental disorder you can think of.

The food industry is using your emotions to control your behavior. That's because they can. They already control your hormones and it's your hormones that control your emotions. Is it any wonder that so many are addicted? Our food industry has done their absolute best to sell you their goods, and that means playing to your emotions in order to sell you that great taste that's going to bring you oh so much discomfort, pain, and disease.

If you had known that this could and would happen to any one of your kids, you'd do everything in your power to change it. You have the power to change it, every time you go to the store. Read the label of everything you buy. If it contains wheat, corn, soy or grains at all, don't buy it. If you do, you'll be buying into a lifetime of pain and discomfort for your family. Choose something else to feed your family. You'll be much further ahead in the long run. The money it will save you in pharmaceuticals is nothing short of astounding. In my estimation, this is criminal behavior. It's criminal behavior being done on an industrial level. Monsanto has politically engineered their control of the FDA and USDA to ensure their compliance in their dominance of our food supply.

Corporate does this on purpose. They do this because they know that we are addicted to our rate of consumption. They also know that with their lobbying power, they can get away with virtually anything. It's the same situation as that of the military-industrial complex. They support congressmen and senators in every state and district, securing their interests, with this influence. Monsanto has even gone to the extent of contracting every farmer that they can, even to the point of suing farmers, just to corner the market. The last corporations that got away with this kind of behavior were busted up by Teddy Roosevelt in the late 19th century. No industry in our history has had more influence on our health, either as an individual or as a society than this grain and sugar industry has with its addictive food. It's created a multi-trillion dollar medical and pharmaceutical industry. The thing that scares them the most is the ketogenic diet as it's the only diet that can save you and the world, from their clutches.

We've allowed these corporations to addict us, worse than we've been any time in the history of man, and that's something for which we should be ashamed. I would be but I didn't set up the Supreme Court to allow Monsanto to patent life in patenting GMO seeds. I didn't even ask them to play with my food supply, yet this toying around with the health of all of their consumers that insist on continuing, bothers me. This may end up being the bane of mankind, as it is a very deadly path for our food industry to be taking. It's one that I consider corporate terrorism.

THE BEST ABOUT THIS DIET REMAINS

THE WAY IN WHICH IT ENDS YOUR PAINS

BY ENDING ALL YOUR INFLAMMATION

FROM STOPPING ALL OF THE GLYCATION

AIDED BY THE GLYPHOSATION

JUST SO YOU'LL NEED MEDICATION

CHAPTER 10

GOD'S ANSWER

The state of our current food supply industry has forced me to reconsider my beliefs in God. It appears that this industry is pure evil with the rampant destruction this industry is content on promoting.

In their quest for profits, they're pulling off quite possibly the most devious deception ever perpetrated on the American people and the world. This can be only be achieved by pure evil or pure greed. My belief is its greed. I don't believe in evil, except for corporate evil, which is another word for greed.

Since greed is a form of evil, I guess we can consider greed, evil. That makes corporate greed, evil is done on an industrial level, or pure evil or as Christians would put it, the devil incarnate. This has forced me to reassess my beliefs in God. I don't believe in God anymore, at least, not the God I was brought up to believe in. That God is too rigid.

I don't believe in a God that is rigid. God is not rigid. Rigid is the antithesis of God. I don't believe in God as much as I live in God. God is not a He or a She as God is not anyone being. God is All Beings, all life either in harmony or discord. God is forever changing along with life and the changing of man. As a man thinks, so thinks God. This idea that God is rigid and never changing, that God is the same today as it was 10,000 years ago or 2000 years ago, is not the faith that Christ taught me. Because I still believe in the Word, I still believe in what Christ taught. What Christ taught is for us to love one another as we love ourselves. I'd like to share how my God works to shape our lives.

Belief in a rigid God is the root of all religious strife, and subsequently most all wars. Most everyone who believes in God believes their God is rigid and never changes. This is how they base their whole set of beliefs, their *isms* wherever their faith takes them, whether they're Catholic, Protestant, Jewish, or Muslim. Their God is a rigid God, One that never changes and who's views never change. It's this attitude of a rigid, never changing the idea of what's sacrosanct, that makes everybody "right by God/Allah" and unwilling to bend and this is what leads to war and terrorism. That's the God I used to worship. I believed in the Word, the Word of Christ.

I still believe in the Word. I just believe as I believe Jesus wanted us to believe, without reservation, without fear and anger, but with Love and Understanding. That is the God I worship but I don't worship a supreme being. What I never realized is, that Word is also my Word. It's also your Word. It's everybody's Word. That is what represents God at any one moment. It's the thoughts and actions and consequences of every living being that comprise Life on earth. That is what God is. It's the good thoughts along with the bad thoughts. This is how God shapes our future, with either thought of Love, the good thoughts or through the god of fear and anger, with bad thoughts.

That puts more importance on our emotions as those are the emotions of God or god. This value of our emotions is regulated, more than anything else, by what we eat and yes carbs do play a part in it. God is different today. God, in Jesus' time, was a god of fear throughout most of the world. But in some civilized parts, there were pockets of civility. These were the villages and towns, where civilization existed and our beliefs of helping and kindness were born. This is also where religion was born.

The people gathering together with common interests were and are the people who make up how God acts and reacts. Whether it is good or bad behavior, it's Us working through God that influences how God operates and how God works. God works through either Love or hate. Is the voice of your God that you hear a Voice of Love or is it a voice of hate?

That, more than anything else dictates what your God is usually like, as God is different at different times. I hope you're beginning to see, your God or god is your inner voice working to tell you how to act and react to each other through god (God). God is Us, All of Us. We(God) work(s) through our inner voices in how we influence each other. This is how God or god works. This is how We work through God (god), whether it be a God of Love or a god of fear and hate.

Therefore God is always moving. God is always changing because of this movement. That means that God is not rigid. God is forever changing just as life changes, constantly and always. That is the forever in God. God is Us, All of Us, together and always changing to meet Our needs. The only quality about God that remains the same is the way in which We work with each other through our emotions. If we can control our emotions, we control God. If we can't control our emotions, god controls us.

The whole point I'm trying to make here is, what controls your emotions, you or your food? The evidence that I've presented in these books is that your diet can control your emotions more than you realize. Carboholics are controlled by their emotions, with their diets and not common sense, whereas ketogenics control their emotions themselves with their diets. The difference is carboholics are controlled by their diet whereas ketogenics control their diet and hence, control their emotions.

That may be why it's easier for us to add the kindness to make life easier. (This comes from our instinct to go back to save our family members while running for our lives from calamity or predators.) This desire to save the family in our Paleolithic days gradually turned into a benevolent civilization when as learned to cultivate wheat. The wheat itself made it malevolent.

God changed at that time. God became more of a God of love instead of just a god of fear. This God of Love's influence grew with the emergence of the church and organized religion. That's also how religions try to control the masses. Most western religions use fear for that control, whereas eastern religions use the consequences of actions cycle or karma, to control the masses.

As this cycle exists today, it controls little to greed for the money, nor does it do much to control the greed for power and it only controls those who fear god. It's the fear of punishment that controls this god, thinking that will prevent the wrongdoing in the first place. By leaving in the god of fear and anger, they're hoping the fear part would easier control the masses. Thus the mantra *"Fear God and you fear nothing else"* was born. This is the foundation of western religions that have a supreme being, like Hebrew, Islam, Christianity, and almost all modern religions, like LDS and Jehovah's Witnesses (two religions based on Christianity except they don't believe in the Trinity).

Being based on Christianity also means that they're based on the Hebrew beliefs about there being a supreme being that controls all. The problem is, there isn't. They don't understand that God isn't 1 rigid supreme being that controls all. God is multiple beings acting unified to create and change our own manifestations in each of our own little worlds. This can completely alter our perception of how God controls our lives because all of us are God if we're united in Love. But then all of us are god as well if we're united in fear.

The question one must ask themselves, in this case, is what God or god do you want to be part of? Do you want a rigid god of fear to control your life or do you want an all-inclusive God of Love, assisting you in that control? This points to why it's important to believe in the God of Love. The God of Love has learned to go past the risk/reward phase of humanity to the *"do it because it's better for humanity"* phase. This is a major step in conquering fear, as it's fear that drives evil. It just happens that fear is driven by hunger. The risk/reward cycle is also driven by hunger.

Many times that's why iniquity happens in the first place. It's the *risk/reward* cycle that promotes it. Too often the risk of achieving the reward is a stronger desire than that of their fear of god (especially when that god doesn't appear to discipline or reward anyone for their actions). This belief can be a fallacy when one doesn't fear god. Without the fear, there's no reason for discipline negating the need for the belief, in turn negating the need for religion. This is the inherent problems with western religions that use this risk/reward cycle for its discipline.

This places much more importance on the diet, as that's the only thing that can replace religion. We've always used the fear of religion to control our emotions, but the real control was from our diet of carbohydrates. Since we've lost that risk/reward cycle that religion used to use to control our emotions, our emotions have gotten out of control. The only way we can truly control them is to control what we eat. This, in turn, gives us control over our hormones and emotions, putting us in control of God instead of a god controlling of us. (Currently, that god is Monsanto and its industries.)

Because most Christians are blind to the real motivation behind any iniquity, they believe them to be acts of God, because their God never changes and he uses these acts as rewards or punishment. Because of he just disciplines and rewards, they're caught trying to solve today's problems, with yesterday's solutions, but their solutions are eons old. They're old as civilization, dating to 2000 years ago, for Christians, 1400 Years for Muslims.

10,000 years for Hebrews (their Bible dates to 10 century BCE). That's about how long each of these religions has existed, all out of the seed of Abraham. The God he Worshiped has become the God of these peoples. It's the very same God worshipped differently in every manner, except one, he is a rigid God in their eyes, one whose ideas never change and this is what directs us all to conflict.

They called the hated god the devil as far back as 9000 years ago. We know now, the hated god isn't the devil, it's us. We are God, so we get to take the responsibility for how our God lives and works within us. This is why we have to protect how we think and work through God. When we create fear, hate, and anger, it drives violence because the only way to fight fear is with anger. Too often it becomes too easy to turn that anger into antagonism and this is where the danger lies. We're experiencing that now. God has all of a sudden turned into an angry god. (I refuse to capitalize the god of hate, as that isn't the God of Love). I believe that God is supposed to be synonymous with Love. That means that God can't hate, as hate has no place in God of Love.

Once all of these religions realize that God is not rigid, but moving, always moving and always changing, that changes Gods perspectives completely. No longer can we ASSUME what God is thinking. What God is thinking and thinking about is always changing, and that will never change. That means that God is forever changing to meet our new and different values and needs. That means that God is never the same God to everyone or everything, nor are God's values and needs to everyone. As man's needs and values change, Gods needs and values change also. How we shape that change only history will tell.

I know what you're thinking, needs? Does God have needs? Uh...yeah. God has needs. The Bible says that God needs our love. That's what the first commandment is, "to Love God with all your heart and mind." If God is all of us, doesn't that mean if we're to love God, we're to love everybody? Isn't that what Jesus was trying to teach us, to love one another as if you love yourself? The point I'm trying to make is that God needs love and that means that We need love because We are God. The Bible says that exactly when it tells us what God's name is. It is I AM. That means that I AM God. That also means that You are God along with everybody else.

As life changes, God changes along with it. God's attitudes change because God is Life. Life forever changes so God forever changes. That changes everything. All of a sudden it's OK to be gay or lesbian, bisexual or transsexual. It's OK to be a different race. None of us are exactly alike as we have to accept the differences in others to be part of a God of Love. God accepts all and loves all. *Accepts*, is the key word here. If God accepts the differences in others, we accept it because we are God and we are always right, because God is always right. That points to your choices, it's your choice to work through a God of Love or a god of hate. Which do you think would make life easier?

God is testing us right now with a possible anti-Christ in the oval office running the free world. An antichrist is a god of hate and our President used a god of hate to promote his candidacy. That makes him a being who uses a god of hate to achieve his goals. This is the definition of an antichrist, one who uses fear and hate to achieve goals of greed and power. This representation of what we see as a god, right now, is full of hate and anger, and he uses that fear and hates to drive the masses into frenzies of anger and antagonism. It's the god of hate that could ruin this country.....and subsequently, the world.

There are those who say they believe in God but deep down inside, they really don't. They think they do but they don't display the traits of someone who truly follows God. They display the traits of someone who follows a god, but only for convenience purposes. They want to believe in the idea of going to heaven because they're afraid of death. They believe in a corporate god, a god of greed and acquisition, a god of possessions and power, not in a God of Love. Those who say they believe in God but really don't, believe this fantasy of God as a punisher or rewarder who's going to rescue them from their iniquities at the end of their mortal lives.

This behavior is also indicative of a carbohydrate diet and the risk/reward cycle, which brings me to my point in this book series. Glucose is an addiction that builds dependence as it makes you hungry, to begin with, and the more you eat, the hungrier you get. That makes this food (which has always been a staple) very dangerous to eat now and stay healthy. Because the hunger cycle is part of the risk/reward cycle, Monsanto's done a very good job of making it very addictive. It's far more addictive now than it's ever been in history.

God being "almighty who controls everything" that watches over us all the time is only partially true. This belief is only partly true, in that God does see everything, but not through one being. God sees everything only because God is everyone. Only all beings can see all things, therefore God cannot be a single being, but multiple beings acting as an entity of its own. That also means that God is not separate from Us. What that means is that only god can separate Us. This also means that God sometimes doesn't recognize god or his actions, elsewhere, due to this erratic behavior that their god creates through its glucose addiction.

Modern Christians believe their God to be a separate supreme being to give them a father figure who can scold them for their iniquities. (All of the iniquities involve greed for money or power of some sort.) Without punishment for wrongdoing, there's no reward for not doing right. This is the basis of our ethics. Some have it. Too many don't.

Christians feel that they should be punished for their evil-doing, not knowing that the evil-doing in itself is going to end up punishing them by the karma their actions generated. If they knew that in the first place, they'd think twice before they acted. Usually, it's greed for money or greed for power that makes people misuse the guidelines that God has given them through the Hebrew Nation on how to treat each other. Instead of treating each other like God asks us to, too many supposedly Christians treat each other with suspicion, fear, and hate. These are the actions of a god of fear and hate and not the God they profess to believe in. This makes most Christians liars by holding onto their belief in a rigid god of fear.

I mentioned that our guidelines or ethics were given to us by a Hebrew god, which is where they come from. All of our values are based on the Ten Commandments from the old testament to the Bible and Torah. These values also show up in the Quran.

(This risk/reward system grew out of our Paleolithic past when running from predators was more important than helping the young or old to keep up with the rest of the group. This is basically what our two-party system has worked out to be, now. One party wants to keep running from the "predators", whereas the other party wants to help those who can't run as fast.) Who's right?

That depends on where your risk/reward cycle plays. Does it play in the carbohydrate domain or does it play in the ketogenic domain? The carbohydrate domain plays with hunger whereas the ketogenic domain doesn't. Hunger may be one of our biggest influences when it comes to greed as hunger is a threat to security.

If one can control their hunger cycle, they have better control of their security, as their hunger can't pose a threat to their security. Most Christians are too wrapped up in their addiction to realize this. Most don't even know that it's the carbs that create and maintain this hunger cycle. This makes the carbs implicit in the iniquity that goes on throughout the world.

Christians need the risk/reward cycle to end their life cycle because of their fear of the unknown. This fear is a direct result of spreading fear and anger throughout their lifetime. All they experience in their own lives, in dealing with God (dealing with everybody in general), is the manner in which they treat other people. The way they treat others is the way in which they will be treated, with either fear and anger or Love. This is how life ends also, with fear or Love.

Those who fear, treat other people with fear. It's what they know best. Often it's the only manner in which they know how to treat each others. It's this treatment or others that's displays, Gods, works within all of us. Those who treat others with Love, Understanding and Respect worship the God of Love. Those who treat others with hate, suspicion, and disdain worship the god of fear and hate. That gives Us the power to manifest how God is going to act and react to any situation. That gives Us the power to be God. Hence We are God.

Once you realize that the unknown is the fullness of God and all God wants is Love, you realize that the unknown is Love, it's a loving embrace of all those who have gone on before us, and when you look at death in that manner, in the same manner, that you treat everyone during life, with love and respect, you discover that there really is nothing at all to fear, except for the fear itself.

That's because of what God needs. The only thing that God needs is our love. God needs it because we need it. The reason most fear death is because they fear to go to hell. Here's a new flash; there is no hell except for what you make. That means that you make your own hell or heaven by the way you influence other people and the impact you've had within the workings of God, day in and day out, throughout your life.

Working with a God of Love leads you to an afterlife of Love. Leading a life of fear, hate and anger are going to lead you to an afterlife of that same fear and hate that you professed your whole life long. What you do throughout your life dictates how your death will manifest itself after you die, so it's your choice what you experience after you die. You can experience Love and all of Gods wonders, or you can experience fear and hate when you die. How you live your life, is what you experience in death. You can expect to see that "on the other side" after you die.

Yet too many old faiths hang on to the traditional reward/punishment cycle and they do this with a rigid God, one that never changes, not even from when man's needs were far from what they are now. They do this to control the faith. That is not the way God works. Instead of the faith controlling the people in my world, the people control the faith. Only in this way can God be forever changing and loving.

But today's religions worship a rigid God, one that never changes, not even from when man's needs were far from what they are now. (That's due to their carb diet, which is as old as civilization.) Their rigid beliefs date back to the cradle of civilization as well, as they still believe strictly, every word in the Bible or Quran, or Torah tells them, about how their faith started and continued until today, never changing.

This has led most foundational and Evangelistic faiths to believe in age-old customs and beliefs that were valid in their time, but they are, no longer. Time is the one thing that God can't control. Time changes everything, as time represents life, forever changing. That means that God can't control the change, only time can. That gives Time power over God because time always changes and makes God change.

If time is more powerful than God, should we worship time or should we just use it as wisely as possible? Maybe that's the best way to worship God. That puts us in control of time, which in turn puts us in control of God. Finally, something that makes sense. That means, we can't *assume* what God wants, as God is us. Saying "what God wants" is code for what that person wants. They just can't take responsibility for saying it themselves, they have to say 'it wants God wants', putting the responsibility on God and not themselves for their choice.

That is one thing we individually have as God, as God has given us that right. It has to do with the right to live. To live you must make choices. Life is nothing but a string of choices, whether good or bad. That is the right to live, the right to make choices. It's those choices we make as God that is written about in the history books of the future. How one's history is written, is dictated by how they live their life. Did they live their lives through a God of Love or a god of fear and hate?

Hence, We are God. You, I, and everyone else in our world, We are All God. We make up what we want to see expressed in God. Whether it's good or bad, it's what we want. And because We are God, We know what God wants, whether good or bad. How we express our will, shows how we want our God to be, whether it's a god of hate or a God of Love. We all live, love-hate and work as God, as God is always moving through us making us make our choices to do such. It's always our choices that make up what God wants, whether we Love it or hate it.

The exciting thing is our world is growing and that means that God is growing. What used to be our whole world 1,000s of years ago was minute compared to today's world. We live in a much bigger world now. (Even though the size of the world hasn't changed, our view of the world and our perspectives have changed. What we see now is much more than what we experienced in the past.) Our world is forever growing. That is the definition of life, the right and ability to grow and as growth means life and life are really Love, that means that growth can only happen through Love. If you want to use fear, hate, and anger, don't expect too much growth.

Will We make God Good, filled with Love? Or will we make god evil, filled with fear, hate, and anger? Which God would you prefer? Would you rather have growth? Or would you rather have stagnation and death? God or god can only manifest their kind of world that we live in. I know which one I want. hate is driven by a carb diet. Love doesn't have to be. All that means is that Love is saner than fear, hate, and anger. Fear hate and anger are driven by cycles of hunger. Love is driven by cycles of inclusion, collaboration and the improvement of our society itself.

As life changes, God changes. God's attitudes change because God is Life. Life forever changes so God forever changes. That really does change everything. Can you believe in a changing God? I do. My God accepts and loves everything and everybody, simply because everybody is God, whether filled with hate and fear or filled with Love. The one filled with Love is much better for your health and thus, much healthier for God and that's why I choose a God of Love to live through. What kind of God/god do you live through?

Do you live through the same corporate god that most people live through? It's a god of greed. It's the god that says he who dies with the most toys wins. Does that sound like a very wise god? It's this god of greed that leads to mistrust of your fellow man and the rest of God that brings on almost all violence, war and terrorism. This makes having anything to do with this god of greed means dealing with mistrust and deceit. That sounds too much like dealing with a god of mistruth and lies. This is not the god of an ethical people. This is the god of people who operate with fear and anger. It's also a god of people addicted to a hunger cycle. This is not the kind of god I want in my world. I can't believe this kind of god. My God isn't that destructive.

I don't believe in god. I Live through God because I am God, at least a part of God. I believe that was Christ's Word that He was trying to spread 2000 years ago and that's why I follow the Word. I believe in the Word, for I am part of the Word. Thank you, Jesus! (Have you ever wondered why we capitalize the first letter of our names like we do God's?)

Sherri always told me to,

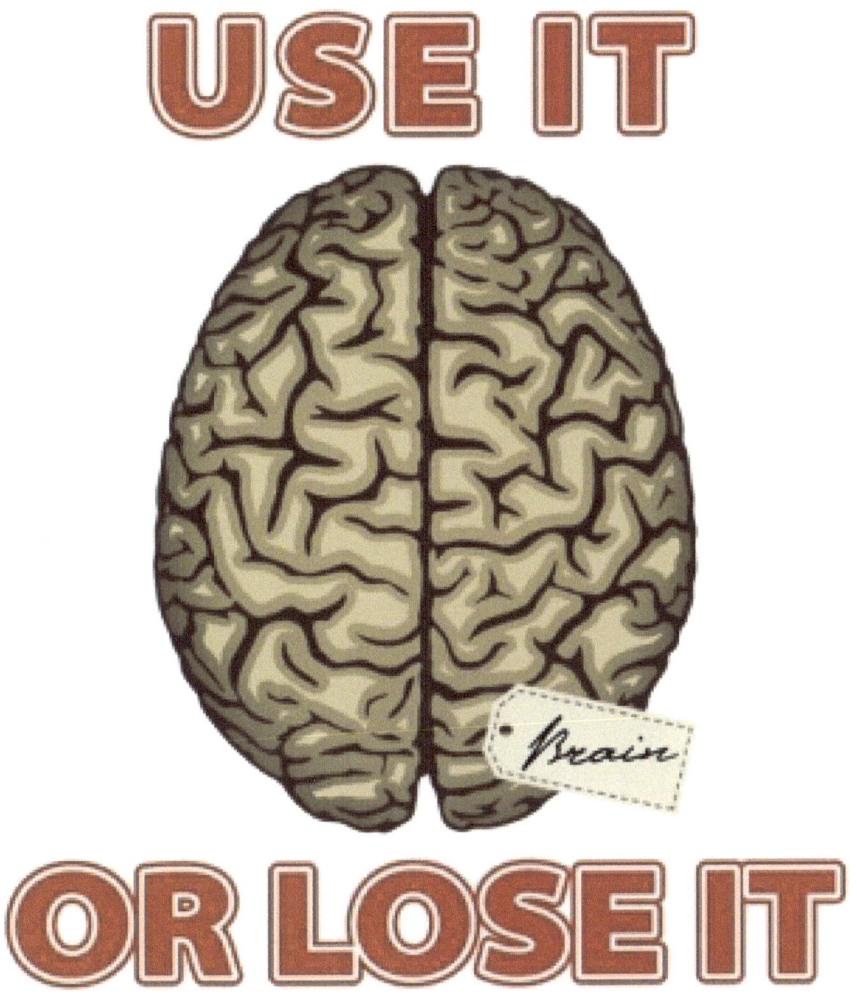

ABOUT THE AUTHOR

3 years ago after suffering from chronic severe pain for 20 years and taking opioids and anti-depressants for the pain, I had to endure 16 of those years, I decided something had to change. On top of the drugs I was taking for pain, I was taking drugs to counteract the side effects of the opioids and anti-depressants and they weren't killing the pain. The pain was always there, I was overweight from the drugs I was taking and I had had enough, I'd tried every form of pain relief that I could find, from acupuncture 2-3 times a week for years at a time, (that was expensive) to TENS treatments to SCENAR therapy to massage therapy to pain blocks (after I had 5 treatments in 5 months, the doctor refused to inject me again, saying that he'd already injected me with too many steroids), yet the blocks worked for about 30 days, then quit, so I had to go back for another. For 4 years I carried an internal nerve stimulator that I'm sure to cost the insurance plenty of money. That thing worked excellently to mask the pain, but it didn't kill it. The pain was always there under the stimulation however the stimulation masked the pain really well. I used that device so much I wore it out after a couple years and had to have it replaced. The SCENAR is the only device that killed the pain but it didn't last much more than one day. That's why I needed a change, so I changed the last thing I could think of changing, my diet. I quit eating bread. Two weeks later and 10 lbs lighter, magic started to happen. Even though It was the toughest thing I've ever had to accomplish, I quit. I ate no more bread, pasta, crackers, tortillas and potato chips and cut way back on the sodas. Actually, I replaced those with juices, which were better at the time, but I've since quit those also. In the last three years, I've modified my diet to a completely ketogenic diet, concentrating my diet on dairy products (milk mostly). I keep my weight at 10 lbs below my prescribed weight and without eating much of anything all day long, I don't get hungry and I don't get sick. That is the largest blessing of a ketogenic diet. Because I can't afford the treatments and the drugs, I stay on my ketogenic diet.

The bonus I get from staying on my keto diet is multiple, no inflammation, less pain and believe it or not, fewer mosquito bites. Due to the lack of glucose flowing through my blood, mosquitoes can't smell it on my breath. They smell acetone on my breath, which means that I don't have glucose in my body. I like that benefit. I can remember times when I had over 70 mosquito bites on my body at any one time. Argh, was that itchy. It's so nice to not have to deal with that now. No glucose was all it took. That in itself is as good a reason as any, to give up your addiction.

PMC report credits:

page 32 credits:
(Eker ET AL., 2006; Bellaloui ET AL., 2009) (Bellaloui ET AL., 2009)

Page 33 credits:
(Nielsen ET AL., 1985; Logan ET AL., 1989; Pricolo ET AL., 1998; Cottone ET AL., 1999; Corrao ET AL., 2001; Green ET AL., 2003) (Ames ET AL., 1993; Coussens & Werb, 2002) *(Lu ET AL., 2013; María ET AL., 1996) (Hernanz & Polanco, 1991)*

page 43 credits:
Hsia TC[1,2], Yin MC[3,4], Mong MC[5].

PMID: 27517907

PMCID: PMC5000686 DOI: 10.3390/ijms17081289 [PubMed - in process] Free PMC Article

page 49 credits:

Nass N1, Ignatov A2, Andreas L3, Weißenborn C2, Kalinski T3, Sel S4.

page 56 credits:
(Broxmeyer, 2002; Díaz-Corrales ET AL., 2004; MacDonald, 2006; Miklossy ET AL., 2006)

Roundup® Trademark of Monsanto - image from Wikipedia.

www.ingramcontent.com/pod-product-compliance
Lightning Source LLC
Chambersburg PA
CBHW041058180526
45172CB00001B/20